THE PATH TO EMPOWERED MASCULINITY

Mastering Strength Sensitivity and Purpose in a Changing World

James A.Smith

TABLE OF CONTENTS

REDEFINING MASCULINITY IN MODERN TIMESH

Masculinity, as a concept, has undergone significant changes over the course of history. In ancient times, masculinity was often defined by physical strength, leadership, and the ability to protect and provide. A man's value was seen largely through his capacity to work, defend his family, and ensure survival. Strength, stoicism, and dominance were key markers of manhood, and these attributes shaped not only societal expectations but also personal identities.

However, as societies developed and cultures evolved, the definition of masculinity expanded. Industrialization, the advent of modern economies, and social movements began to alter the nature of gender roles. The expectations placed on men to be solely providers and protectors started to shift as women's roles in the workforce expanded and traditional household dynamics evolved.

This shift has only accelerated in recent decades. Today, the idea of masculinity is far more complex than it has ever been. It is no longer confined to the stereotypes of aggression, dominance, and emotional repression. Men are encouraged to embrace their sensitivity, express their emotions, and be nurturing, which contrasts with the historical ideals of rugged stoicism and impenetrable strength.

Yet, this evolving picture of masculinity can be confusing for many men. The modern world often sends mixed messages:

Be strong but sensitive; be assertive but humble; be driven but not domineering. This creates internal tension as men seek to balance expectations from the past with the evolving values of the present.

The struggle to reconcile these shifts in masculinity has left many men questioning their place in the world. What does it mean to be a man in today's society? What values should one uphold? How do you navigate the fine line between strength and sensitivity without losing your sense of self? These are not just questions of social adaptation; they are deeply personal and existential challenges that many men face in the modern age.

The Pressure of Modern Masculinity

While traditional masculinity placed clear, albeit rigid, expectations on men, the modern era presents a unique set of challenges. The pressure to "have it all" – career success, emotional availability, financial security, and personal fulfillment – can be overwhelming. On top of this, the fast-paced digital world, with its social media-driven comparisons and cultural shifts, has intensified the pressure.

In many cultures, men are still expected to maintain a sense of emotional stoicism, often driven by the belief that vulnerability is a weakness. As a result, many men struggle with expressing their emotions, fearing that they might be perceived as weak or overly sensitive. However, suppressing emotions can lead to a wide range of psychological issues, from anxiety and depression to anger and frustration, further complicating a man's sense of identity.

Compounding this issue is the pervasive culture of success, which equates a man's worth with his achievements, financial status, and ability to excel in competitive environments. While ambition is an admirable trait, when combined with unrelenting societal expectations, it can lead to burnout, stress, and feelings of inadequacy.

The Need for a New Definition of Strength

For generations, strength has been a central pillar of traditional masculinity. However, the definition of strength needs to evolve. Physical strength and toughness are no longer the sole attributes that define a man's ability to be strong. Instead, strength today can be seen in one's ability to remain emotionally present, to persevere in the face of adversity, and to nurture meaningful relationships.

True strength now lies in balancing confidence with humility, and ambition with empathy. A man who is truly strong is one who can stand firm in his beliefs while also allowing himself to be vulnerable. It's about taking responsibility for one's actions, embracing accountability, and striving for growth— not just in the professional or material sense but also in the emotional and spiritual realms.

The world no longer needs men who are stoic pillars of emotional isolation. Instead, it calls for men who are brave enough to connect with their emotions, who can express their fears and weaknesses without shame, and who understand that strength is not the absence of vulnerability but the courage to embrace it. This new version of strength fosters deeper connections with others, leading to healthier relationships, more resilient families, and communities built on trust and understanding.

Sensitivity as a Strength

In modern society, sensitivity is often misunderstood as a weakness, particularly for men. But sensitivity, when properly embraced, is a profound strength. It allows men to better understand and connect with the emotions of others, fostering empathy, compassion, and genuine relationships.

Sensitivity does not mean being overly emotional or reactive. Instead, it is the capacity to be aware of one's emotions, recognize the emotions of others, and respond thoughtfully rather than impulsively. In a world that increasingly values emotional intelligence, sensitivity is becoming a critical skill for men who want to build strong, authentic relationships in both personal and professional settings.

For many men, however, embracing sensitivity requires breaking through layers of conditioning that have taught them to suppress their feelings. From a young age, boys are often told to "toughen up" or "stop crying," which instills the belief that emotions are something to be ashamed of. Undoing this conditioning requires intentional effort, self-reflection, and sometimes external support. But the reward is immense: men who embrace their sensitivity become more self-aware, emotionally balanced, and capable of fostering deeper connections with others.

The journey to mastering modern masculinity is not a one-size-fits-all process. It involves embracing both strength and sensitivity, recognizing the unique challenges that modern men face, and forging a path that aligns with one's values and purpose. This means not only meeting external expectations but also cultivating an internal sense of fulfillment.

In a world that is constantly evolving, men must redefine their sense of purpose and identity in ways that are authentic, sustainable, and emotionally fulfilling. Purpose, in this sense, is about more than career achievements or societal success. It's about living in alignment with one's true self, understanding what brings meaning and joy, and using that understanding to positively impact others.

By mastering the balance between strength and sensitivity, and by reclaiming a sense of purpose in a rapidly changing world, men can step into a new era of empowered masculinity. One that honors the past, embraces the present, and builds a future where both men and the people around them thrive.

SOCIETAL SHIFTS AND THEIR IMPACT ON MEN'S IDENTITIES

Over the past century, society has undergone profound changes that have redefined cultural norms, social expectations, and the roles that men are expected to play. These shifts have directly impacted how men perceive themselves, how they interact with others, and how they navigate their personal identities. Understanding these changes is critical for men who seek to balance the competing demands of traditional expectations with modern realities.

The Decline of Traditional Gender Roles

Historically, men's identities were closely tied to traditional gender roles. Men were expected to be the breadwinners, the protectors, and the decision-makers, while women often took on caregiving roles in the family and community. These clear distinctions between male and female roles provided a blueprint for manhood that was rigid, yet easily understood. Masculinity was primarily measured by a man's ability to work, provide, and lead.

However, starting in the 20th century, the world began to change in ways that blurred these gender distinctions. The feminist movements, particularly during the 1960s and 1970s, challenged the notion that women should be relegated to the private sphere. As more women entered the workforce, sought higher education, and gained greater political and social influence, the need for men to adjust their roles became apparent. Traditional masculinity began to clash with these new dynamics, forcing men to reconsider what it meant to be a provider and protector when women were also taking on those responsibilities.

The decline of rigid gender roles opened up new possibilities for both men and women but also created uncertainty. Men who were raised with the belief that their value lay in their ability to provide or dominate found themselves questioning their purpose in a world where those expectations were less relevant. Many men now face the challenge of redefining their roles within relationships, families, and society at large.

The Impact of Economic Shifts on Masculinity

Economic shifts have played a significant role in the transformation of masculine identity. The industrial age that defined the 19th and early 20th centuries placed a premium on physical labor and manufacturing jobs, which were dominated by men. These jobs provided a clear avenue for men to assert their masculinity through hard work, discipline, and the ability to provide for their families.

However, as the global economy shifted towards technology, information, and service-based industries, the traditional male-dominated fields began to decline. This economic transition has been particularly challenging for men in working-class communities, where job loss in manufacturing industries has created a sense of dislocation and loss of purpose. As manual labor jobs declined, men were increasingly required to enter fields that may not align with traditional masculine ideals of physical strength or independence.

This shift has led to an identity crisis for many men. The sense of self-worth that came from having a stable, well-paying job has been eroded. Economic instability has affected men's ability to provide for their families in the way their fathers and grandfathers did, leading to feelings of inadequacy or failure. This has particularly impacted men in regions where job opportunities in traditional industries are scarce, creating long-term psychological and emotional challenges.

Changing Family Structures

The changes in family dynamics over the last several decades have also significantly impacted men's identities.

Divorce rates have risen, single-parent households have become more common, and non-traditional family structures such as cohabitation or blended families are now widespread. The traditional nuclear family, with a male breadwinner and a stay-at-home mother, is no longer the dominant model.

These shifts in family structures require men to adapt to new roles within the family unit. Many men now find themselves as primary caregivers, sharing responsibilities in raising children and managing household tasks in ways that were uncommon in previous generations. The rise of stay-at-home dads is one example of how family roles are evolving.

While this evolution allows men to form deeper, more nurturing relationships with their children and partners, it can also challenge deeply ingrained societal beliefs about masculinity. Some men struggle with feelings of emasculation or societal judgment when they take on roles traditionally associated with women. This creates internal tension, as the desire to be a loving, engaged father conflicts with cultural norms that still place value on a man's ability to work and provide.

Furthermore, the dissolution of the nuclear family has brought about the challenge of maintaining masculinity within the context of co-parenting, step-parenting, or managing relationships post-divorce. Men must learn how to navigate these complex emotional and social terrains while still retaining a sense of their identity.

The Influence of Feminism and Gender Equality Movements

The feminist movement and the push for gender equality have been critical in reshaping how men and women relate to each other. Feminism's advocacy for women's rights, equal pay, reproductive rights, and freedom from gender-based discrimination has been instrumental in achieving greater gender equity. However, this progress has also required men to reevaluate their own roles, power dynamics, and privileges.

For many men, the feminist movement has brought about a welcome opportunity to shed the burden of hypermasculine expectations. Feminism encourages men to embrace vulnerability, share their feelings, and engage in equitable partnerships, all of which promote healthier relationships and well-being.

However, for other men, the rise of feminism has been perceived as a threat to their traditional understanding of masculinity. Some men feel displaced by the advancement of women in professional and social arenas, and this sense of displacement can foster resentment or confusion. Men who feel uncertain about how to balance their own aspirations with the push for greater gender equality may struggle to find their place in a world that is rapidly changing.

The challenge is to recognize that gender equality is not a zero-sum game. The liberation of women from traditional gender roles also frees men from the confines of toxic masculinity. By embracing equality, men have the opportunity to redefine their relationships, careers, and identities in ways that are more emotionally fulfilling and balanced.

Media and Pop Culture's Role in Shaping Modern Masculinity

In recent years, the media and pop culture have played an increasingly powerful role in shaping perceptions of masculinity. From television shows and movies to advertisements and social media, the portrayal of men has shifted from the archetype of the stoic, unemotional hero to a more diverse and complex representation.

Contemporary media often celebrates men who defy traditional norms. Men who openly express vulnerability, nurture relationships, and value emotional intelligence are increasingly visible in popular culture. Celebrities, athletes, and influencers who advocate for mental health awareness, gender equality, and emotional wellness are helping to reshape the narrative around what it means to be a man in modern times.

However, this shift is not without its challenges. While some media platforms celebrate more progressive forms of masculinity, others continue to promote hypermasculine ideals, glorifying aggression, material success, and dominance over others. Social media, in particular, can contribute to toxic comparisons as men are bombarded with images and messages about how they should look, act, and succeed. The pressure to conform to unrealistic standards of masculinity can lead to insecurity, anxiety, and disconnection from one's true self.

As society continues to evolve, men have the opportunity to reclaim an authentic sense of masculinity that aligns with their values and emotions. This process requires introspection and a willingness to challenge outdated cultural norms. By embracing both strength and sensitivity, acknowledging the impact of societal shifts, and navigating the complexities of modern life with integrity, men can forge a new path forward.

This new masculinity doesn't reject the past entirely, nor does it conform blindly to modern expectations. Instead, it allows men to define themselves on their terms—balancing ambition with emotional awareness, independence with community, and tradition with progress. By doing so, men can not only improve their own lives but also contribute to a more inclusive, compassionate society.

BREAKING FREE FROM LIMITING STEREOTYPES

For generations, men have been boxed into rigid stereotypes that define how they should behave, feel, and relate to others. These stereotypes often emphasize traits such as toughness, emotional stoicism, dominance, and independence, leaving little room for vulnerability, emotional expression, or the embrace of qualities traditionally viewed as "feminine." The pressure to conform to these limiting ideals can be suffocating, leading to internal conflict and feelings of inadequacy for many men. Breaking free from these stereotypes is not only essential for personal growth and well-being but also for creating more authentic, meaningful relationships with others.

To understand how to break free from limiting stereotypes, it's important to first explore their origins. Many of the stereotypes surrounding masculinity date back centuries, rooted in social structures that relied on clear gender roles for survival. In hunter-gatherer societies, for example, men were often expected to be protectors and providers, roles that required physical strength, aggression, and emotional resilience. Over time, these qualities became synonymous with what it meant to be a man.

As society evolved, these gender roles became more entrenched, reinforced by religious institutions, cultural traditions, and legal frameworks. Men were expected to be heads of households, leaders in their communities, and the primary earners, while women were relegated to caregiving roles. This division of labor reinforced the idea that men must be strong, unemotional, and dominant—traits that were believed to be essential for their success.

Even in modern times, media, literature, and popular culture have continued to perpetuate these stereotypes. Movies, TV shows, and advertisements often depict men as heroes who solve problems through violence or assertiveness, while emotional vulnerability is portrayed as a sign of weakness. This cultural messaging has created a narrow definition of masculinity, one that leaves little room for men to fully express themselves without facing judgment or ridicule.

The Psychological Toll of Conforming to Stereotypes

The pressure to conform to limiting masculine stereotypes can take a significant psychological toll on men. Many men internalize the belief that they must always be strong and in control, even when faced with difficult emotions or life challenges. This leads to emotional repression, where men feel unable or unwilling to express their true feelings for fear of appearing weak or vulnerable. Over time, this emotional suppression can lead to serious mental health issues such as depression, anxiety, and anger.

For some men, the pressure to conform to masculine ideals can also manifest in destructive behaviors. Aggression, substance abuse, and risky behaviors are often seen as ways to assert one's masculinity, especially in cultures that glorify hypermasculinity. However, these behaviors often mask deeper emotional pain and only serve to perpetuate the cycle of self-destructive patterns. In essence, the stereotype of "toughness" becomes a prison, limiting men's ability to seek help or engage in self-reflection.

Additionally, the demand to conform to traditional stereotypes often leads men to struggle with interpersonal relationships. Men may find it difficult to connect emotionally with partners, children, or friends because they've been conditioned to view emotional intimacy as incompatible with masculinity. The result is often loneliness, dissatisfaction, and strained relationships—outcomes that further reinforce the stereotype that men must "go it alone."

Redefining Strength and Emotional Vulnerability

One of the most effective ways to break free from limiting stereotypes is to redefine what it means to be strong. Traditional notions of strength are often tied to physical prowess, emotional detachment, or the ability to dominate others. However, true strength comes from being able to balance emotional resilience with emotional vulnerability. Strength is not the absence of fear or pain, but the ability to confront those feelings, process them, and emerge with a deeper understanding of oneself.

In this context, emotional vulnerability should be seen as a strength rather than a weakness. Men who are willing to acknowledge and express their feelings—whether it be sadness, fear, or joy—are better equipped to navigate life's challenges and build meaningful connections with others. Vulnerability allows for emotional growth, self-awareness, and greater empathy, all of which are crucial for personal development and healthy relationships.

Furthermore, breaking free from stereotypes requires men to expand their definition of masculinity to include a wider range of traits. Compassion, collaboration, and nurturing should not be viewed as traits exclusive to women but as human qualities that are essential for everyone. By embracing these qualities, men can develop a more balanced and holistic sense of self.

The Role of Media and Culture in Breaking Stereotypes

Media and culture play a powerful role in both reinforcing and challenging stereotypes. In recent years, there has been a noticeable shift in the portrayal of masculinity in popular media. Films, TV shows, and advertising campaigns are increasingly featuring men who defy traditional masculine ideals. These portrayals include men who are stay-at-home dads, men who openly express their emotions, and men who champion gender equality.

While this shift is encouraging, there is still much work to be done. Media can continue to play a transformative role by creating more diverse representations of masculinity that reflect the complexity of modern men's experiences. Men should be encouraged to explore their full range of emotions and talents, without being confined to outdated notions of what it means to be a man.

It's also essential for men to critically engage with the media they consume. Being aware of how certain portrayals of masculinity can influence behavior is the first step in rejecting limiting stereotypes. Men can seek out and support content that offers a broader vision of masculinity, one that includes emotional complexity, vulnerability, and equality.

How to Break Free: Practical Steps

Breaking free from limiting stereotypes requires both introspection and action. Here are some practical steps men can take to redefine their sense of masculinity:

1. Self-Reflection: Men need to take the time to reflect on their beliefs about masculinity and where those beliefs come from. Are these beliefs serving their well-being, or are they holding them back? Self-awareness is the key to identifying and breaking down limiting stereotypes.

2. Embrace Emotional Expression: Men should allow themselves to feel and express their emotions freely. Whether through journaling, talking to a trusted friend, or seeking therapy, emotional expression is crucial for mental health and personal growth.

3. Challenge Cultural Norms: It's important for men to challenge societal expectations that promote toxic masculinity. This can include calling out harmful behaviors in their social circles, supporting gender equality, and embracing qualities like empathy and collaboration.

4. Seek Support: Men shouldn't feel they have to navigate the process of breaking stereotypes alone. Whether through friendships, support groups, or mental health professionals, seeking help and sharing experiences can be incredibly empowering.

5. Redefine Success: Men should expand their definitions of success beyond traditional measures like wealth, status, or physical strength. Success can also be measured in terms of emotional fulfillment, meaningful relationships, and personal authenticity.

Breaking free from limiting stereotypes is not just about rejecting old ideals—it's about building a new, more empowering vision of masculinity. Men have the opportunity to create a sense of self that embraces both strength and sensitivity, independence and connection. By letting go of rigid expectations, men can lead fuller, more authentic lives, free from the pressure to conform.

Ultimately, breaking these stereotypes is about reclaiming the freedom to define masculinity on one's own terms. Men can craft identities that reflect their true selves, rather than the outdated ideals of the past. In doing so, they not only improve their own lives but also contribute to a world where men and women alike can thrive without the burden of limiting expectations.

STRENGTH AND VULNERABILITY

For centuries, strength has been synonymous with physical power, dominance, and control. The image of the "strong man" has often been tied to muscularity, aggression, and an unshakable emotional fortitude. However, in today's world, this narrow definition of strength is being challenged by a more holistic understanding—one that values emotional depth, vulnerability, and self-awareness. Strength, in its true form, is not about suppressing emotions or dominating others; it's about finding the balance between resilience and openness. This chapter will explore how strength and vulnerability, when embraced together, form a new and empowering power dynamic for men.

Redefining Strength: Beyond Physicality

Traditionally, strength has been viewed through the lens of physical power. The ability to lift heavy weights, endure physical hardship, or protect others through sheer force has been praised as the ultimate expression of masculinity. While physical strength is undoubtedly a valuable trait, it is only one dimension of what it means to be strong. True strength transcends the physical; it encompasses emotional resilience, mental toughness, and the ability to adapt and grow in the face of life's challenges.

In modern society, where emotional intelligence and interpersonal skills are becoming increasingly important, the ability to navigate one's emotions and connect with others has emerged as a critical aspect of strength. Men who are in touch with their emotions are better equipped to handle stress, build meaningful relationships, and face adversity with grace and composure. Strength, in this sense, is not about suppressing feelings, but about recognizing and harnessing them in a way that promotes personal growth and emotional well-being.

Emotional strength, like physical strength, requires training. Just as one might go to the gym to build muscle, men must engage in emotional work to develop their capacity for vulnerability, empathy, and self-reflection. This doesn't make them weaker; on the contrary, it makes them more adaptable, resilient, and capable of leading fulfilling lives. Embracing a broader definition of strength allows men to be more well-rounded, authentic, and ultimately, more powerful.

The Courage to Be Vulnerable

Vulnerability is often seen as the opposite of strength, particularly in traditional views of masculinity. The idea that men should "man up" and hide their emotions is deeply ingrained in many cultures, leading to a widespread belief that showing vulnerability is a sign of weakness. However, this outdated mindset ignores the fact that vulnerability requires immense courage. Opening up to others, admitting fears, and facing one's insecurities are acts of bravery that demand a great deal of inner strength.

When men allow themselves to be vulnerable, they open the door to deeper connections and personal growth. Vulnerability fosters trust in relationships, as it allows others to see the real person behind the facade of toughness. By sharing their struggles and fears, men can create space for empathy, understanding, and mutual support, whether in romantic partnerships, friendships, or professional environments.

Moreover, vulnerability is essential for personal development. It enables men to confront their limitations, learn from their mistakes, and seek help when needed. In a world that often pressures men to have all the answers, vulnerability provides the freedom to admit that no one has everything figured out. This openness to learning and growth is a sign of true strength because it reflects the ability to evolve and adapt in response to life's challenges.

The Strength in Asking for Help

One of the greatest misconceptions about strength is that it requires complete self-reliance. Many men feel that asking for help is a sign of weakness or failure, leading them to shoulder burdens alone, even when doing so is detrimental to their well-being. However, recognizing when to seek support is a hallmark of strength, not weakness.

Asking for help demonstrates self-awareness—the ability to recognize one's limitations and understand that no one can do everything alone. Whether it's reaching out to a friend for emotional support, consulting a mentor for guidance, or seeking therapy to work through mental health struggles, asking for help is an act of wisdom and strength. It takes courage to admit that you don't have all the answers and that sometimes, the strongest thing you can do is lean on others.

In this new power dynamic, strength is not about going through life solo but about building a network of support. Men who embrace vulnerability and ask for help are more likely to thrive in their personal and professional lives because they understand the value of collaboration and connection. This ability to rely on others when needed, while also offering support in return, creates a balanced and sustainable approach to navigating life's challenges.

Strength and Empathy: Building Stronger Connections

Another key aspect of this new understanding of strength is empathy—the ability to understand and share the feelings of others. While empathy has often been associated with femininity, it is a crucial trait for men to develop as well. Empathy strengthens relationships by fostering understanding and compassion, allowing men to connect with others on a deeper level.

In the context of masculinity, empathy is a powerful tool for breaking down barriers and overcoming stereotypes. Men who practice empathy are better equipped to navigate conflicts, resolve misunderstandings, and support those around them. Whether in personal relationships, the workplace, or within broader societal contexts, empathetic men can create environments of trust and collaboration, rather than competition and isolation.

Empathy also plays a critical role in self-compassion. Men who are empathetic towards themselves are more likely to practice self-care, forgive themselves for mistakes, and approach challenges with a growth mindset. This internal empathy strengthens emotional resilience, allowing men to bounce back from setbacks and maintain a positive outlook even in difficult times.

Balancing Strength and Vulnerability

The idea that strength and vulnerability are mutually exclusive is a myth that has limited men for far too long. In reality, the two are deeply interconnected, and it is only by embracing both that men can unlock their full potential. Strength without vulnerability leads to emotional repression, isolation, and burnout. Vulnerability without strength can result in a lack of boundaries and an inability to cope with life's difficulties. The balance between these two forces creates a new, more dynamic form of power—one that allows men to be both resilient and open, both tough and compassionate.

In this new power dynamic, men are free to define their own sense of masculinity based on their unique strengths and values. They are no longer confined to outdated ideals of what it means to be a man, but are empowered to embrace their full range of emotions and capabilities. By finding this balance, men can build healthier relationships, achieve personal fulfillment, and lead with confidence in a changing world.

As society continues to evolve, so too must our understanding of masculinity. Strength and vulnerability are not opposites, but complementary traits that, when balanced, create a powerful and authentic sense of self. Men who embrace this new power dynamic are not only better equipped to navigate their own emotional landscapes but are also more likely to thrive in their relationships, careers, and communities.

THE IMPORTANCE OF EMOTIONAL VULNERABILITY FOR PERSONAL GROWTH

Emotional vulnerability, often misunderstood as weakness, is in fact one of the most powerful tools for personal growth. In a world that frequently encourages emotional stoicism, especially in men, embracing vulnerability is an act of courage and self-awareness. It is the willingness to open oneself up to uncertainty, discomfort, and emotional exposure, which can feel risky but is essential for true transformation and connection. Emotional vulnerability is not about being fragile or passive, but about being authentic in the face of life's challenges. It allows for deep personal insight, builds resilience, and fosters healthier relationships with oneself and others.

Vulnerability as a Path to Self-Awareness

One of the key benefits of emotional vulnerability is the heightened self-awareness it brings. When we allow ourselves to be vulnerable, we are no longer hiding behind emotional defenses or societal expectations. Instead, we confront our true feelings—our fears, insecurities, desires, and aspirations. This process can be uncomfortable, as it forces us to face parts of ourselves that we may have previously ignored or repressed. However, by acknowledging these emotions, we gain a deeper understanding of who we are.

Vulnerability helps us identify the areas in our lives where we need to grow. For example, admitting that we feel inadequate or anxious in certain situations can lead to valuable insights about where we may lack confidence or need to develop new skills. Without vulnerability, these feelings often remain hidden beneath the surface, preventing us from addressing them and moving forward. By being open about our emotions, we unlock the potential for real change and self-improvement.

Overcoming Fear and Building Resilience

At the core of emotional vulnerability is the willingness to confront fear—whether it's the fear of rejection, failure, or being judged by others. Many people avoid vulnerability because they are afraid of these outcomes, preferring instead to maintain a facade of invulnerability. However, this avoidance comes at a cost. By shutting down emotionally, we limit our potential for personal growth, stifle our creativity, and hinder our ability to form meaningful connections with others.

Embracing vulnerability requires acknowledging and confronting these fears, but in doing so, we build resilience. Each time we allow ourselves to be vulnerable—whether by sharing our feelings, taking a risk, or admitting our mistakes—we grow stronger. We learn that vulnerability does not lead to disaster but rather opens the door to growth and new opportunities. As we become more comfortable with vulnerability, our fear diminishes, and we become more capable of handling life's uncertainties.

Resilience is built not by avoiding challenges but by facing them head-on. Emotional vulnerability teaches us to embrace discomfort as a natural part of the growth process. It shows us that setbacks and failures are not permanent but are simply stepping stones toward personal development.

Over time, this mindset shift helps us become more adaptable, confident, and emotionally strong.

Deepening Relationships Through Vulnerability

Another crucial aspect of emotional vulnerability is its role in deepening relationships. Authentic connections with others are rooted in vulnerability. When we allow ourselves to be emotionally open, we give others the opportunity to see who we truly are, beyond the surface-level persona. This openness fosters trust and intimacy, which are the foundations of meaningful relationships.

In many relationships, both personal and professional, there is a tendency to maintain emotional distance in order to protect oneself from being hurt or rejected. However, this emotional guardedness creates barriers that prevent genuine connection. By contrast, when we show vulnerability—by expressing our emotions, sharing our struggles, or admitting when we need help—we invite others to do the same. This mutual vulnerability creates a sense of safety and understanding, allowing relationships to flourish.

In romantic relationships, vulnerability is especially important. Being vulnerable with a partner allows for deeper emotional intimacy, which strengthens the bond between individuals. It enables partners to understand each other's emotional needs, support each other through difficult times, and build a relationship based on mutual trust and empathy. Without vulnerability, relationships often become superficial, lacking the emotional depth needed to thrive over the long term.

In friendships and professional relationships, vulnerability can also be transformative. Being open about one's emotions, challenges, and limitations can lead to greater collaboration, mutual respect, and a stronger sense of community. Vulnerability breaks down walls and encourages authentic communication, which leads to more meaningful and productive interactions.

Vulnerability and Personal Growth

The connection between vulnerability and personal growth is profound. When we embrace vulnerability, we open ourselves up to new experiences, learn from our mistakes, and become more self-aware. Vulnerability challenges us to step outside of our comfort zones and take risks, which is essential for personal development. It pushes us to confront our fears, acknowledge our limitations, and strive for continuous improvement.

For instance, in a professional context, vulnerability might mean admitting when we don't know something or asking for feedback from colleagues. While this may feel uncomfortable, it creates opportunities for learning and growth. Similarly, in our personal lives, being vulnerable might involve acknowledging our need for emotional support, seeking therapy, or working on personal issues that we've been avoiding. These actions, though difficult, are essential for personal transformation.

In addition, vulnerability fosters creativity and innovation. When we allow ourselves to take risks and explore new ideas without fear of failure, we unlock our creative potential. Many of the world's most successful individuals attribute their achievements to their willingness to be vulnerable—whether by pursuing unconventional paths, experimenting with new ideas, or embracing the possibility of failure.

Reframing Vulnerability as Strength

The societal narrative often portrays vulnerability as a weakness, particularly for men. From a young age, many are taught to suppress their emotions, avoid showing weakness, and maintain an image of invulnerability. This mindset, however, is detrimental to personal growth and emotional well-being. In reality, vulnerability is not a sign of weakness but a display of strength. It takes immense courage to be vulnerable, to show the world who you truly are, and to take emotional risks.

When we reframe vulnerability as a strength, we begin to see it as an essential component of a fulfilling life. Vulnerability allows us to grow, connect, and thrive. It helps us become more emotionally resilient, self-aware, and capable of navigating life's complexities. By embracing vulnerability, we take control of our personal growth and unlock the potential for deeper relationships, greater self-understanding, and a more fulfilling life.

Emotional vulnerability is not a liability but a powerful tool for personal growth. It requires courage, self-awareness, and resilience to open oneself up to emotional discomfort and uncertainty, but the rewards are immense. Vulnerability leads to greater self-understanding, deeper relationships, and the strength to face life's challenges with confidence and grace. By embracing emotional vulnerability, individuals can break free from limiting societal norms, experience profound personal growth, and create a more authentic and fulfilling life.

EMOTIONAL INTELLIGENCE AND SENSITIVITY

In today's complex and interconnected world, emotional intelligence (EQ) has emerged as a critical skill that enhances success in both personal and professional relationships. While traditional concepts of masculinity have often emphasized strength, decisiveness, and self-reliance, modern masculinity is beginning to recognize the value of emotional intelligence and sensitivity. These traits allow individuals to navigate the emotional landscapes of life with greater depth, empathy, and understanding. Far from being a sign of weakness, emotional intelligence is a powerful strength that can foster deeper connections, healthier relationships, and a more balanced life.

Defining Emotional Intelligence

Emotional intelligence refers to the ability to recognize, understand, and manage both your own emotions and the emotions of others. It involves several key components:

1. Self-awareness: The ability to recognize and understand your own emotions, as well as how they affect your thoughts, behaviors, and interactions with others. Self-awareness is the foundation of emotional intelligence, as it enables individuals to be in touch with their emotional state and to understand how their feelings influence their actions.

2. Self-regulation: The ability to control or redirect disruptive emotions and impulses. This involves staying composed under pressure, managing emotional responses in a

constructive way, and maintaining a level of emotional balance.

3. Motivation: Emotional intelligence involves being motivated not only by external rewards but by internal goals and values. High-EQ individuals are driven by a sense of purpose, and they are able to maintain a positive attitude even in the face of setbacks.

4. Empathy: The ability to understand and share the feelings of others. Empathy allows individuals to step into someone else's shoes, to appreciate their perspective, and to respond in a compassionate and supportive way.

5. Social skills: This involves the ability to manage relationships effectively, to communicate clearly, and to work collaboratively with others. Emotional intelligence helps individuals navigate the social dynamics of life with ease, fostering cooperation, trust, and mutual respect.

Emotional Intelligence: A Critical Skill for Success

While traditional IQ measures cognitive intelligence, EQ is equally—if not more—important for success in life and relationships. High emotional intelligence allows individuals to handle interpersonal relationships judiciously and empathetically, which is essential for success in both personal and professional settings.

In the workplace, for instance, emotional intelligence plays a key role in leadership, team collaboration, conflict resolution, and decision-making. Leaders with high emotional intelligence are better able to inspire, motivate, and support their teams. They are skilled at managing their own emotions, which enables them to stay calm and composed in high-pressure situations, and they are adept at reading and responding to the emotions of others, which fosters trust and loyalty among team members.

In personal relationships, emotional intelligence is equally crucial. It allows individuals to navigate the emotional complexities of intimate relationships with greater understanding and empathy. Emotionally intelligent individuals are better able to communicate their feelings, listen to their partner's needs, and respond with compassion. This leads to healthier, more fulfilling relationships that are based on mutual respect, trust, and emotional support.

The Connection Between Emotional Intelligence and Sensitivity

Sensitivity is often viewed negatively in traditional masculine paradigms, as it is sometimes associated with vulnerability or emotional fragility. However, sensitivity, when combined with emotional intelligence, becomes a hidden strength. Being sensitive to the emotions of others is a key aspect of empathy, which is a cornerstone of emotional intelligence.

Sensitive individuals are often highly attuned to the feelings and needs of those around them. This ability to pick up on emotional cues and respond with care is a valuable skill in both personal and professional contexts. In relationships, sensitivity allows individuals to recognize when their partner is upset or in need of support, even when the other person may not express it directly. This fosters deeper emotional connections and strengthens the bond between partners.

In the workplace, sensitivity enables leaders to understand the emotional dynamics of their teams, which can help them manage conflicts, boost morale, and create a more inclusive and supportive work environment. Rather than being a liability, sensitivity is a strength that enhances emotional intelligence and enables individuals to connect with others on a deeper level.

How Emotional Intelligence and Sensitivity Empower Men

For men, embracing emotional intelligence and sensitivity requires a shift in mindset. Traditional notions of masculinity often emphasize stoicism, self-reliance, and emotional suppression. Men are frequently taught to "toughen up," avoid showing vulnerability, and handle challenges on their own. However, this approach can lead to emotional isolation, strained relationships, and increased stress. By contrast, developing emotional intelligence allows men to experience a more holistic and balanced form of masculinity—one that incorporates strength with emotional depth, decisiveness with empathy, and self-reliance with meaningful connections.

1. Building deeper relationships: Emotional intelligence fosters the development of healthier and more authentic relationships. When men are emotionally intelligent, they are better able to express their emotions in a way that is clear and constructive, which helps prevent misunderstandings and conflicts in relationships. Moreover, they are more attuned to the emotions of others, which enables them to be more supportive, compassionate partners, friends, and family members.

2. Reducing stress and anxiety: Emotional suppression can lead to a buildup of stress, frustration, and anxiety. Men who embrace emotional intelligence and sensitivity are better equipped to manage their emotions and deal with stress in a healthy way. They are able to identify and address their emotional needs, seek support when necessary, and avoid the emotional burnout that often results from trying to "go it alone."

3. Enhancing leadership and collaboration: In professional settings, emotional intelligence is a key factor in effective leadership. Leaders who are emotionally intelligent are better able to inspire and motivate their teams, manage conflicts, and create a positive and productive work environment. Men who develop emotional intelligence are not only more effective leaders but also more collaborative team members, as they are able to navigate social dynamics with greater ease and empathy.

4. Promoting personal growth and self-awareness: Emotional intelligence is a critical component of personal growth. It allows men to develop a deeper understanding of their emotions, motivations, and desires. This self-awareness leads to greater emotional maturity, better decision-making, and a more fulfilling life. By embracing their sensitivity and emotional intelligence, men can unlock their full potential and achieve a greater sense of purpose and fulfillment.

Emotional intelligence and sensitivity are not weaknesses—they are hidden strengths that can enhance success in every aspect of life. By developing emotional intelligence, men can build deeper relationships, reduce stress, enhance their leadership abilities, and promote personal growth. Sensitivity, when combined with emotional intelligence, allows individuals to connect with others on a deeper level, fostering empathy, compassion, and understanding.

In a world that increasingly values emotional intelligence, men who embrace their emotional sensitivity and develop their emotional intelligence are not only breaking free from limiting stereotypes but also unlocking their full potential for personal and professional success. Emotional intelligence is the key to thriving in modern life and relationships, and it is a vital component of empowered masculinity.

PRACTICES FOR DEVELOPING EMOTIONAL INTELLIGENCE AND SENSITIVITY

Emotional intelligence (EQ) and sensitivity are essential skills that can be developed through intentional practices and self-awareness. These traits not only enhance personal well-being but also foster deeper relationships and improve professional success. Below are practical strategies for cultivating emotional intelligence and sensitivity in everyday life, along with detailed explanations on how each practice contributes to growth.

1. Self-Reflection and Awareness

The foundation of emotional intelligence lies in self-awareness, which is the ability to recognize and understand your own emotions, thoughts, and reactions. Cultivating self-awareness requires regular self-reflection, where you examine your feelings, behaviors, and the underlying reasons behind them.

How to Practice Self-Reflection:

- Journaling: Keeping a daily or weekly journal helps you track your emotional responses to various situations. Writing down how you feel and why you felt that way can illuminate patterns in your emotional life that you might not have noticed before. Journaling encourages introspection and provides clarity on how emotions influence your decisions and behaviors.
- Mindful moments: Throughout the day, take short pauses to check in with yourself. Ask, "What am I feeling right now?" and "Why am I feeling this way?" Becoming aware of your emotional state in real-time helps you manage your reactions, especially during stressful situations.

Self-reflection strengthens your ability to recognize emotional triggers and to understand how your emotions shape your actions. Over time, this practice fosters emotional maturity and helps you respond to life with greater emotional control and intention.

2. Active Listening to Enhance Empathy

Empathy, one of the core components of emotional intelligence, is the ability to understand and share the feelings of others. Developing empathy requires a conscious effort to listen actively and attentively during conversations. Active listening goes beyond simply hearing words; it involves fully engaging with the speaker, both verbally and non-verbally.

How to Practice Active Listening:

- Give undivided attention: When someone is speaking to you, put away distractions like your phone or other tasks. Maintain eye contact and nod or offer small verbal affirmations to show that you're fully present.
- Focus on understanding, not responding: Often, we listen with the intention of crafting a reply rather than truly understanding the other person. Practice listening without interrupting or thinking about what you will say next. Focus entirely on the speaker's words and emotions.
- Ask clarifying questions: To deepen your understanding of the other person's emotions, ask questions like, "How did that make you feel?" or "Can you tell me more about that experience?" This shows that you are interested in their emotional experience and that you value their perspective.

Active listening fosters stronger relationships by showing others that you care about their feelings. It also enhances your ability to understand others' emotions, which improves both personal and professional interactions. The more empathetic you become, the more sensitive you will be to the needs of those around you.

3. Emotional Regulation Techniques

Managing your own emotions is another key aspect of emotional intelligence. Emotional regulation involves controlling and modifying your emotional responses in order to avoid impulsive reactions and maintain emotional balance. This practice allows you to stay calm under pressure and handle challenging situations with grace.

How to Practice Emotional Regulation:

- Deep breathing exercises: When you feel overwhelmed by emotions like anger, frustration, or anxiety, take a few moments to focus on your breath. Slow, deep breathing helps activate the parasympathetic nervous system, which calms your body and mind. Inhaling for four counts, holding for four, and exhaling for four can be a quick way to regain composure.
- Cognitive reappraisal: This involves changing the way you think about a situation in order to alter your emotional response. For example, if someone criticizes your work, instead of reacting defensively, reframe the criticism as an opportunity for growth. Shifting your perspective can reduce negative emotional reactions and encourage a more constructive mindset.
- Practice gratitude: Cultivating a habit of gratitude can shift your focus away from negative emotions. When you find yourself spiraling into frustration or stress, pause to think about something positive in your life. Regularly practicing gratitude can create a more optimistic emotional baseline, helping you stay emotionally grounded.

Emotional regulation leads to greater resilience and mental clarity. It prevents emotional outbursts, reduces stress, and allows you to respond to challenges in a composed and rational manner. Mastering emotional regulation can also improve your relationships, as it demonstrates emotional maturity and reliability.

4. Mindfulness and Meditation

Mindfulness is the practice of staying present in the moment, fully aware of your thoughts, feelings, and surroundings without judgment. Meditation is a structured form of mindfulness that trains your mind to focus and become more aware of your emotions. Both mindfulness and meditation help improve emotional intelligence by enhancing self-awareness, emotional regulation, and empathy.

How to Practice Mindfulness and Meditation:

- Mindfulness during daily activities: Instead of letting your mind wander during routine tasks, like eating or walking, focus on the sensations, sounds, and emotions associated with those activities. For example, notice the taste and texture of your food as you eat or feel the rhythm of your footsteps as you walk. This practice trains your brain to stay present and connected to your emotions.
- Guided meditation: Apps or online resources provide guided meditations that help you focus on your breath, body, or emotions. Start with short sessions of 5 to 10 minutes and gradually increase the duration as you become more comfortable. Regular meditation helps calm the mind and builds your ability to manage your emotions effectively.
- Body scan meditation: This practice involves mentally scanning your body from head to toe, noticing areas of tension or discomfort. By paying attention to physical sensations, you can become more attuned to how emotions manifest in your body, which increases emotional awareness.

Mindfulness and meditation improve your ability to stay present and fully experience your emotions without becoming overwhelmed by them. These practices reduce anxiety and stress, improve focus, and enhance empathy. Over time, mindfulness creates a more balanced emotional life and increases your overall sense of well-being.

5. Building Healthy Relationships Through Vulnerability

Embracing emotional vulnerability is essential for developing emotional intelligence. Many men, due to societal pressures, may shy away from vulnerability, seeing it as a sign of weakness. However, vulnerability is a key ingredient for building trust, intimacy, and deeper connections in relationships.

How to Practice Vulnerability:

- Share your feelings openly: In your close relationships, make a conscious effort to share your thoughts and emotions. This might involve expressing fears, insecurities, or concerns that you might otherwise keep hidden. Vulnerability builds trust and invites others to do the same, leading to more authentic connections.
- Admit when you need help: Asking for help is a vulnerable act that many people resist, especially in a culture that values independence. However, recognizing when you need support—whether emotional or practical—and reaching out to others is a strength. It shows self-awareness and humility, both important aspects of emotional intelligence.

- Acknowledge mistakes: Owning up to mistakes requires emotional courage and vulnerability. Whether in your personal or professional life, acknowledging where you went wrong and taking responsibility fosters a culture of trust and respect. It also demonstrates emotional maturity and promotes growth.

By practicing vulnerability, you allow others to see you more fully, which deepens trust and fosters emotional intimacy. Vulnerability is key to developing more authentic relationships and enhancing your emotional intelligence.

6. Empathy Development Through Volunteering and Social Interaction

Another powerful way to cultivate emotional intelligence is by placing yourself in environments that challenge you to understand and empathize with others. Volunteering and engaging in social activities that involve diverse groups of people expand your perspective and build your capacity for empathy.

How to Practice Empathy in Social Settings:

- Volunteer for community service: Engaging in volunteer work allows you to encounter people from different walks of life, often facing challenges that you may not personally experience. This exposure broadens your understanding of human emotions and helps develop your ability to empathize with others' struggles.
- Participate in group activities: Joining social or professional groups that involve collaboration can help you practice empathy. Whether it's a book club, sports

team, or networking group, engaging with others in shared activities helps you better understand different personalities, emotional responses, and perspectives.

Engaging in social and volunteer activities fosters greater empathy by exposing you to diverse emotional experiences. It also strengthens your social skills and emotional intelligence by requiring you to navigate various interpersonal dynamics.

FINDING PURPOSE

In today's fast-paced, ever-evolving world, many men struggle to connect with a deeper sense of purpose. With societal expectations shifting, traditional roles changing, and external pressures intensifying, it's easy to feel lost, unsure of your direction, or disconnected from what truly drives you. Yet, discovering your inner purpose isn't just about fulfilling society's expectations—it's about finding what makes you feel alive, motivated, and authentic. Let's guide you through understanding your purpose, the importance of self-discovery, and how you can tap into that inner drive to lead a more fulfilled and empowered life.

What is Purpose, and Why Does It Matter?

Purpose is the internal compass that guides your decisions, fuels your passion, and gives meaning to your actions. It's the unique mission that defines who you are beyond your roles in society, relationships, or career. A strong sense of purpose offers more than just direction—it provides motivation, resilience, and a deeper sense of fulfillment.

Many people mistakenly believe that purpose must be something grand or world-changing, like becoming a leader, philanthropist, or entrepreneur. While those goals are admirable, your purpose can also be deeply personal and connected to small, meaningful acts in everyday life. Whether you aim to make a positive difference in your community, create art, or be a supportive partner and father, your purpose is valid and significant as long as it resonates with your inner self.

The Inner Journey: How to Begin Discovering Your Purpose

Discovering your purpose requires a commitment to self-exploration, vulnerability, and reflection. Below are practical steps you can take to uncover your true mission and reconnect with what drives you:

1. Reflect on What Brings You Joy and Fulfillment

One of the most effective ways to uncover your purpose is by identifying the activities, people, and experiences that make you feel truly alive. Purpose often emerges from the things that bring you the most joy or the moments when you feel a sense of fulfillment.

Ask yourself questions like:

- What do I love to do, even when no one is watching?
- When do I feel most energized and engaged?
- What moments in life have made me feel deeply fulfilled?

These questions help you identify patterns in your life that may point to your deeper purpose. For instance, if you feel most fulfilled when helping others solve problems, your purpose may involve serving others, mentoring, or coaching.

2. Examine Your Strengths and Talents

Another way to find purpose is to assess your natural strengths and talents. What are the skills or abilities that come easily to you? What do others often praise you for? Your unique strengths offer clues to your purpose, as they reveal how you can contribute to the world in meaningful ways.

Reflect on your personal talents:

- Are you a natural leader who brings people together?
- Are you a great listener who helps others feel understood?
- Do you have a creative talent or technical skill that you're passionate about developing?

Purpose often lies at the intersection of what you're good at and what the world needs. By aligning your strengths with a cause, mission, or activity that matters to you, you can create a purposeful path.

3. Revisit Childhood Dreams and Passions

As children, we often have a clear sense of what excites us and what we're passionate about. Over time, societal expectations, responsibilities, and the pressure to "fit in" can cause us to suppress those dreams. Reconnecting with your childhood interests and passions can help you tap into your true desires and motivations.

Ask yourself:

- What did I want to be when I was younger, before I was told what I "should" be?
- What hobbies or interests did I have that made me lose track of time?
- Have I abandoned a passion that once brought me joy?

Revisiting these dreams may reignite a sense of purpose that has been dormant for years. Even if your childhood aspirations seem impractical now, they can provide insights into your core values and what truly matters to you.

4. Identify the Problems You Want to Solve

Purpose often arises from a desire to address challenges or issues that resonate with you personally. Many people find their mission in life by dedicating themselves to causes or problems they feel passionate about solving. Whether it's environmental conservation, social justice, mental health advocacy, or community building, focusing on a specific cause can give your life direction.

Consider these questions:

- What societal or global issues upset me the most?
- Which injustices or challenges am I passionate about addressing?
- What do I believe the world needs more of?

If there is a specific problem or cause that stirs your heart, consider how your skills, passions, and strengths can contribute to solving it. Purpose-driven individuals often find that contributing to the greater good gives their lives more meaning and fulfillment.

Overcoming Barriers to Discovering Your Purpose

Finding purpose isn't always easy, and it's normal to encounter challenges along the way. Whether it's self-doubt, fear of failure, or pressure from external sources, you may struggle with identifying or pursuing your mission. Below are some common barriers to finding purpose and strategies to overcome them:

- Fear of Judgment or Rejection: Many people hesitate to pursue their purpose because they fear being judged or rejected by others. This fear often stems from societal expectations or a desire to fit in. To overcome this, remind yourself that your purpose is personal and unique to you. It doesn't need to conform to others' standards. Stay true to what fulfills you, even if others don't understand it.
- Perfectionism: Some individuals become paralyzed by the belief that their purpose must be perfectly clear or that they need to have it all figured out. In reality, purpose is something that evolves over time. Rather than waiting for everything to be perfect, take small steps toward what excites and inspires you. Purpose often becomes clearer through action, not contemplation.
- Distractions and External Pressures: In today's busy world, it's easy to get caught up in daily responsibilities, distractions, and societal pressures that pull you away from discovering your true purpose. To combat this, carve out intentional time for reflection, meditation, or journaling. Prioritizing moments of quiet and solitude allows you to reconnect with your inner voice and focus on what matters most.

Living with Purpose: How Purpose Transforms Your Life

Once you've identified your purpose, it becomes a guiding force that influences every area of your life. Purpose creates a sense of alignment, where your thoughts, actions, and decisions are all moving in the same direction. This sense of direction gives your life greater meaning and fulfillment, even in the face of challenges.

Purpose is a powerful motivator that drives you to wake up every morning with enthusiasm. It gives you the resilience to overcome obstacles and the clarity to make decisions that align with your core values. Purpose can also help you maintain a positive mindset, as it encourages you to focus on the bigger picture rather than getting lost in daily frustrations.

When you live with purpose, you also become more aware of the impact you have on others and the world around you. Purpose-driven individuals often find that their actions, no matter how small, contribute to something greater than themselves. This sense of contribution fosters deep satisfaction and a lasting sense of fulfillment.

Finding purpose is not a one-time event—it's a lifelong journey of self-discovery, growth, and alignment. As you move through different phases of life, your purpose may evolve, expand, or shift. However, by staying connected to your inner self and remaining open to new experiences, you can continue to refine and deepen your sense of purpose.

Your personal mission and purpose are what make you uniquely you. Embrace the process of discovering your purpose with curiosity, patience, and dedication. As you do, you'll unlock new levels of strength, fulfillment, and empowerment that will guide you through every stage of life.

ALIGNING YOUR CAREER AND GOALS WITH A DEEPER SENSE OF PURPOSE

One of the most fulfilling aspects of living with purpose is when your career and personal goals align with your deeper sense of meaning. It's one thing to discover your inner purpose, but integrating that purpose into your everyday work and long-term ambitions can transform your life on a profound level. When your career and goals reflect your personal mission, you experience a sense of harmony and authenticity, where every action contributes to a larger vision that resonates deeply with who you are.

Understanding Purpose in the Context of Work and Ambition

Work plays a significant role in most people's lives, taking up a large portion of time and mental energy. However, many individuals feel disconnected from their jobs, seeing work as a means to an end rather than a pathway toward fulfillment. This is where the alignment between purpose and career becomes vital. Your purpose gives your work direction, passion, and meaning, making it more than just a source of income—it becomes a platform for you to express your values, skills, and contributions to the world.

When you align your career with purpose, you're not simply going through the motions to meet societal expectations or pay the bills. Instead, you're living in accordance with your values, driven by a larger vision that excites you and challenges you to grow.

How to Begin Aligning Your Career with Purpose

1. Reflect on Your Core Values and Passions

The first step in aligning your career with purpose is to identify your core values. These are the principles that define who you are and what matters most to you. Whether it's creativity, innovation, service, community, or personal growth, your values guide the choices you make in life. A career that aligns with your values will naturally bring a greater sense of satisfaction and meaning.

Ask yourself:

- What principles do I hold dear in my personal life?
- What type of impact do I want my work to have on others or the world?
- What activities make me feel fulfilled and in tune with myself?

Once you have clarity on your values, examine whether your current career supports or hinders them. If your work environment or daily tasks conflict with your values, you may need to reassess your career path or make adjustments to bring it into alignment with your purpose.

2. Define Your Personal Mission

Your personal mission is the unique way you intend to contribute to the world, and it's closely tied to your purpose. Once you've clarified your core values, consider how those values translate into a broader mission that can guide your career decisions. Your mission might be to inspire others through creative expression, to promote social justice, to solve complex problems, or to provide care and support to those in need.

Reflect on your personal mission by asking:

- What is the unique contribution I want to make to the world?
- How can I use my skills, experiences, and passions to make a difference?
- In what areas of life or work do I feel called to create positive change?

Your mission will serve as a guiding light, helping you make career choices that align with what matters most to you. It will also provide you with resilience when challenges arise, as you'll know that your efforts are part of a larger purpose.

3. Consider How Your Current Career Fits Into Your Purpose

If you're already working in a particular field, the next step is to assess how well your current career aligns with your sense of purpose. While it may not be possible for every job to perfectly match your mission, there are often ways to shift your approach or role to better reflect your purpose. Sometimes, this might involve seeking out new opportunities within your current organization, such as moving into leadership, mentoring, or advocacy roles that align with your values.

Evaluate your current role by asking:

- Does my work bring me a sense of fulfillment and satisfaction?
- Do I feel that my job allows me to make a positive impact?

- Are there ways to reshape my responsibilities or focus to better align with my purpose?

If your current career doesn't reflect your purpose, don't be afraid to explore new paths. A career shift doesn't necessarily mean starting over—it can mean pivoting toward opportunities that align more closely with your values.

4. Explore Purpose-Driven Career Paths

For those who feel a strong disconnect between their current career and personal purpose, exploring purpose-driven career paths may be necessary. This could involve researching industries or professions that are more closely aligned with your mission. For example, if your purpose revolves around helping others, you might explore careers in social work, healthcare, or education. If you're driven by creativity, you might pursue opportunities in art, design, or entrepreneurship.

To explore new career paths, consider:

- What industries or roles would allow me to express my core values?
- How can I leverage my skills and talents to contribute to a cause or mission I care about?
- Are there opportunities for me to align my work with my personal mission, either through volunteer work or side projects?

Sometimes, aligning your career with purpose doesn't require a complete overhaul of your professional life. Instead, you can start by taking small steps, such as pursuing passion projects, volunteering, or seeking out purpose-driven roles within your current industry.

Setting Purposeful Goals for Career Growth

In addition to aligning your career with your purpose, it's essential to set personal and professional goals that reflect your mission. Purposeful goals give your career direction and ensure that your efforts are moving you toward something meaningful. When setting goals, consider both short-term and long-term objectives that reflect your desire for growth, fulfillment, and contribution.

1. Set Goals That Align with Your Core Values

When setting career goals, start by making sure they reflect your core values. For example, if community service is important to you, set a goal to incorporate community engagement into your work. If creativity is your passion, your goals might include developing new skills or starting a creative project that excites you.

Ask yourself:

- Does this goal reflect my values and purpose?
- How will achieving this goal contribute to my overall mission in life?
- What steps can I take to ensure that my professional growth aligns with my personal mission?

2. Prioritize Growth and Contribution

Purpose-driven goals aren't just about personal success— they're about making a positive impact. When setting goals, think about how your growth can benefit others. Whether it's mentoring, leading by example, or contributing to a cause, your goals should reflect your desire to make a difference.

Ask yourself:

- How can I use my skills to benefit others?
- What opportunities can I create that will have a positive impact on my community or industry?

3. Create a Roadmap for Purposeful Achievement

Once you've identified your purposeful goals, create a roadmap for achieving them. This roadmap should include both the practical steps needed to reach your goals and the emotional and mental mindset required to stay focused on your mission. Purposeful achievement requires persistence, resilience, and a commitment to your values, even in the face of setbacks.

Ask yourself:

- What steps do I need to take to align my career with my purpose?
- How can I stay motivated and connected to my mission, even when challenges arise?
- What support or resources will help me on this journey?

MASCULINITY AND MENTAL HEALTH

In modern times, the conversation about mental health has gained significant momentum, but the subject of men's mental health still remains heavily stigmatized. Historically, men have been socialized to view emotions as a sign of weakness, and societal expectations of masculinity have often discouraged open discussions about mental health struggles. This toxic culture of silence has contributed to high rates of depression, anxiety, and suicide among men, with many suffering in silence because they feel that seeking help is a sign of failure.

However, it is crucial to break the silence around men's mental health challenges. The traditional image of men as stoic, unemotional beings no longer serves the complex reality of modern life. More than ever, men need to develop the tools to address their emotional and mental well-being, and that starts by dismantling the stigma associated with mental health struggles.

The Relationship Between Masculinity and Mental Health

Traditional masculine ideals have long been associated with traits like strength, resilience, independence, and stoicism. These traits, while admirable in certain contexts, can become barriers to emotional expression and mental health support. Men are often conditioned to believe that they must handle problems on their own, never show vulnerability, and "tough it out" when facing emotional difficulties. These outdated beliefs reinforce a sense of isolation and prevent men from reaching out when they need help the most.

This creates a troubling cycle: men, feeling the pressure to conform to these ideals, suppress their emotional struggles, leading to further mental distress. Instead of seeking help, many turn to unhealthy coping mechanisms like substance abuse, aggression, or emotional withdrawal. The fear of being perceived as weak or unmanly becomes a significant obstacle, and this suppression of emotions can contribute to more severe mental health issues over time.

The Stigma of Seeking Help

One of the most damaging aspects of the stigma around men's mental health is the belief that seeking help is a sign of weakness. From an early age, boys are often taught to "man up" and not express their emotions. This conditioning leads many men to internalize the idea that they should be self-reliant in all areas of life, including mental health. As a result, the act of seeking professional help or even opening up to friends or family can feel like a failure of their masculinity.

The stigma attached to therapy, counseling, or mental health services further compounds the issue. Men are less likely than women to seek help for mental health problems, and when they do, it's often much later, when symptoms have worsened or reached a crisis point. This reluctance to seek help is deeply rooted in cultural attitudes and the fear of judgment from peers and society at large.

But seeking help is not a sign of weakness—it's an act of courage. Reaching out for support, whether through therapy, support groups, or simply talking to someone, is a powerful step toward healing and growth. Mental health issues are not a reflection of a person's strength or value; they are part of the human experience. Breaking the stigma involves challenging these ingrained beliefs and recognizing that everyone, including men, deserves support and care when facing mental health challenges.

Recognizing the Signs of Mental Health Struggles

To address the stigma surrounding men's mental health, it's essential for men to be able to recognize the signs of mental health struggles, both in themselves and in others. Mental health issues manifest differently in men, and the symptoms are often masked by behaviors that don't immediately signal emotional distress.

For many men, depression or anxiety may not show up as overt sadness or worry. Instead, it can appear as irritability, anger, or withdrawal. Men may also turn to workaholism, over-exercising, substance abuse, or risky behaviors as a way to cope with their emotions. Recognizing these patterns of behavior is a key step in acknowledging that something deeper may be at play.

Common signs of mental health struggles in men include:

- Emotional numbness: Feeling disconnected from one's emotions or unable to express how one feels.
- Increased irritability or anger: Frustration or anger that seems disproportionate to the situation.
- Withdrawal from social activities: Avoiding friends, family, or social events.
- Substance abuse: Using drugs or alcohol as a means to cope with emotional distress.

- Workaholism or excessive exercise: Using work or physical activity to avoid confronting emotional issues.
- Sleep disturbances: Insomnia or sleeping too much as a way to escape emotional pain.

By understanding these symptoms, men can begin to take action, rather than letting their struggles go unnoticed or untreated.

Encouraging Emotional Expression and Vulnerability

One of the most important shifts in addressing men's mental health is encouraging emotional expression and vulnerability. In many cultures, men are taught to suppress their feelings, often out of fear that showing vulnerability will make them appear weak or inferior. However, vulnerability is not a weakness—it's an essential aspect of emotional health and human connection.

Men must be encouraged to share their emotions, whether it's with a trusted friend, partner, or therapist. Creating spaces where men feel safe to express their feelings is crucial. Support groups, mental health awareness campaigns, and conversations about emotional well-being can help dismantle the belief that men should always be strong and emotionless.

It's important to recognize that vulnerability is a form of strength. It takes courage to admit that you're struggling and to seek help. When men are open about their emotional challenges, they not only help themselves but also contribute to a broader cultural change that destigmatizes mental health for everyone.

The Role of Therapy and Support Systems

Therapy plays a vital role in helping men confront and overcome mental health challenges. Counseling provides a safe, nonjudgmental space where men can explore their emotions, identify patterns of behavior, and develop healthier coping mechanisms. Therapy can also help men dismantle the rigid beliefs about masculinity that have been ingrained in them and redefine what it means to be strong and resilient.

Building a strong support system is equally important. Whether through friends, family, or community groups, having people to talk to and rely on is a critical aspect of mental health. For many men, developing deeper emotional connections with others can be a transformative experience. When men feel supported and understood, they are more likely to open up about their struggles and seek help when needed.

Support systems also help break the cycle of isolation that many men experience. By normalizing conversations about mental health, men can build stronger connections with others and reduce the stigma surrounding emotional vulnerability.

As we move toward a more progressive understanding of masculinity, it's essential to continue breaking down the stigma around men's mental health. Modern masculinity should embrace the full range of human emotions, including vulnerability, fear, sadness, and joy. Men should be empowered to express their feelings without fear of judgment or shame.

Breaking the silence around mental health doesn't just benefit individual men—it benefits society as a whole. When men are emotionally healthy and supported, they are better equipped to contribute to their relationships, families, and communities. Healthy masculinity involves embracing the complexity of emotions and acknowledging that mental health is just as important as physical health.

The path to empowered masculinity includes breaking the stigma around mental health. Men must be encouraged to acknowledge and address their emotional struggles, seek support, and embrace vulnerability as a strength rather than a weakness. By challenging outdated beliefs about masculinity, we can create a world where men feel free to prioritize their mental well-being without fear of judgment.

Empowered masculinity means taking ownership of one's mental health, building strong support systems, and embracing the power of emotional resilience. When men break free from the silence, they open the door to healing, growth, and deeper, more fulfilling connections with themselves and others.

PRACTICAL WAYS TO SEEK HELP AND BUILD RESILIENCE

Addressing mental health challenges and building resilience are crucial steps in the path toward empowered masculinity. Men often face societal pressure to handle emotional struggles on their own, but seeking help is a powerful act of self-care that leads to personal growth. Resilience, on the other hand, is the ability to recover from difficulties and adapt in the face of adversity. By taking practical steps to prioritize mental health, men can build emotional strength and maintain balance in their lives.

1. Acknowledge and Accept Your Emotions

The first step in seeking help and building resilience is acknowledging and accepting your emotions. Many men are conditioned to suppress their feelings, whether it's sadness, anxiety, frustration, or fear. However, suppressing emotions only compounds the problem, making it harder to process and manage them. Acknowledging emotions allows you to understand what you're feeling, why you're feeling that way, and what action you need to take to address it.

To practice this, start by regularly checking in with yourself. Set aside a few minutes each day to reflect on how you feel, without judgment. Journaling can be a helpful tool for this process, allowing you to express your thoughts and emotions on paper. By recognizing your emotional state, you can take the first step toward healing.

2. Reach Out to Trusted Friends and Family

One of the simplest but most powerful ways to seek help is by reaching out to trusted friends or family members. Sharing your thoughts and feelings with people who care about you creates a sense of connection and support. While it might feel uncomfortable at first, expressing vulnerability strengthens relationships and helps combat feelings of isolation.

You don't need to have all the answers or solutions to your problems when talking to someone. Simply opening up about how you feel can be a relief in itself. It can also serve as a reminder that you're not alone and that there are people in your life who want to support you through difficult times.

When choosing whom to confide in, select individuals who have shown empathy, patience, and understanding in the past. These are the people most likely to offer a safe, nonjudgmental space for you to express yourself.

3. Consider Professional Help: Therapy and Counseling

While talking to friends and family can provide valuable emotional support, seeking professional help from a therapist or counselor offers a structured and effective way to address deeper issues. Therapy is not a sign of weakness but a proactive step toward healing and growth. Mental health professionals are trained to help you navigate complex emotions, identify patterns of thought and behavior, and develop coping strategies.

Therapy provides a safe, confidential space to explore issues that may be difficult to discuss with others. Whether you're dealing with stress, anxiety, depression, or unresolved trauma, a therapist can help guide you toward better mental health. Cognitive Behavioral Therapy (CBT), for example, is a popular approach that helps individuals challenge negative thought patterns and develop healthier ways of thinking.

If you're unsure where to start, consider reaching out to your healthcare provider, researching online therapy platforms, or asking for recommendations from people you trust.

4. Join a Support Group or Community

Support groups offer a unique environment where individuals facing similar challenges come together to share their experiences, provide encouragement, and offer advice. Joining a support group for men's mental health can be incredibly empowering, as it helps break down the stigma surrounding emotional vulnerability. In these spaces, men can feel less isolated, knowing that others have gone through similar struggles.

Whether in person or online, support groups create a sense of belonging and understanding that can be difficult to find elsewhere. Group members offer different perspectives on coping with challenges, and hearing others' stories can inspire hope and resilience.

For those interested in men-specific groups, organizations like Movember, Man Therapy, or HeadsUpGuys provide resources and community spaces dedicated to men's mental health.

5. Engage in Regular Physical Activity

Physical health and mental health are deeply interconnected. Engaging in regular physical activity can have a profound impact on your emotional well-being. Exercise stimulates the production of endorphins—chemicals in the brain that act as natural mood boosters. It also helps reduce stress, anxiety, and symptoms of depression.

Incorporating physical activity into your routine doesn't require you to spend hours at the gym. Even simple activities like walking, running, cycling, or yoga can make a significant difference. The goal is to find an activity that you enjoy and can commit to regularly.

Additionally, physical activity often serves as a form of mindfulness, allowing you to focus on the present moment and temporarily distance yourself from worries or stressors.

6. Develop a Resilience-Building Mindset

Resilience isn't about avoiding challenges; it's about developing the capacity to navigate and bounce back from them. Building resilience involves shifting your mindset to focus on growth and learning rather than feeling overwhelmed by setbacks. Here are some practical ways to foster a resilience-building mindset:

- Embrace Challenges as Opportunities for Growth: Instead of viewing difficulties as insurmountable obstacles, try to see them as opportunities to learn and grow. When you encounter a challenge, ask yourself, "What can I learn from this situation?" This shift in perspective can help reduce the fear and anxiety associated with adversity.
- Practice Self-Compassion: Treat yourself with the same kindness and understanding that you would offer a friend. It's easy to be critical of yourself when things go wrong, but self-compassion allows you to move through tough times with greater ease. Acknowledge that everyone makes mistakes and that failure is a natural part of life.
- Focus on What You Can Control: During times of stress or uncertainty, it's common to feel overwhelmed by factors outside of your control. Instead, focus on what you

can influence and take small, actionable steps to improve your situation. This approach helps you regain a sense of agency and reduces feelings of helplessness.

- Cultivate Gratitude: Regularly practicing gratitude helps shift your focus from negative experiences to positive aspects of your life. It can be as simple as writing down three things you're grateful for each day. Over time, this practice can foster a more optimistic outlook, which contributes to greater resilience.

7. Set Healthy Boundaries

Setting and maintaining healthy boundaries is a crucial component of building resilience. Boundaries help protect your mental and emotional well-being by preventing burnout, reducing stress, and ensuring that you have the time and energy to care for yourself.

Boundaries can be physical, emotional, or time-related. For instance, limiting work-related tasks outside of working hours, saying no to social engagements when you need rest, or choosing to disengage from toxic relationships are all forms of boundary-setting.

By setting boundaries, you create space for self-care and prioritize your needs. Boundaries also foster healthier relationships, as they allow you to engage with others in a way that respects both your limits and theirs.

8. Practice Mindfulness and Meditation

Mindfulness and meditation are powerful tools for managing stress and building emotional resilience. These practices involve paying attention to the present moment without judgment and can help you become more aware of your thoughts and feelings.

Mindfulness helps reduce rumination on past events or anxieties about the future, allowing you to stay grounded in the here and now. It can also increase self-awareness, making it easier to recognize emotional triggers and respond to them in a healthy way.

Incorporating even a few minutes of meditation or mindfulness practice into your daily routine can have a positive impact on your mental health. There are many apps and resources available to guide you through mindfulness exercises, such as Headspace or Calm.

9. Maintain a Balanced Routine

Resilience comes from creating balance in all aspects of life—work, rest, and play. A balanced routine ensures that you're taking care of your mental, emotional, and physical health. Prioritize activities that bring you joy and relaxation, such as spending time with loved ones, pursuing hobbies, or practicing self-care.

By establishing routines that prioritize both productivity and relaxation, you create a sustainable lifestyle that supports long-term resilience. When life becomes stressful, having a balanced routine in place helps you manage pressure more effectively.

10. Celebrate Small Wins

Finally, don't underestimate the importance of celebrating your progress, no matter how small it may seem. Building resilience is an ongoing process, and recognizing the steps you've taken to improve your mental health reinforces positive behavior. Celebrate each milestone, whether it's reaching out for help, practicing self-care, or overcoming a particular challenge. This acknowledgment helps build confidence and reinforces your ability to cope with future difficulties.

In conclusion, seeking help and building resilience are essential steps in living a mentally healthy and fulfilling life. By developing emotional awareness, reaching out for support, and fostering a growth mindset, men can overcome challenges and thrive in both their personal and professional lives. Empowered masculinity includes not only physical strength but also emotional resilience, self-care, and the courage to seek help when needed.

CULTIVATING A MINDSET OF GROWTH AND SELF-COMPASSION

Developing a mindset of growth and self-compassion is one of the most transformative practices for personal development. It empowers you to view challenges as opportunities, build resilience in the face of adversity, and treat yourself with kindness when things don't go as planned. For men navigating the complexities of modern masculinity, this shift is essential in fostering emotional well-being and embracing long-term success.

What is a Growth Mindset?

A growth mindset is the belief that your abilities, intelligence, and talents can be developed through dedication, learning, and effort. Coined by psychologist Carol Dweck, the concept emphasizes that people aren't born with fixed traits. Instead, with the right attitude, they can continually evolve, improve, and achieve new goals.

For many men, the pressure to succeed often leads to a fixed mindset, where they believe that their worth is determined by innate talent or performance in specific areas like work, physical strength, or social status. This belief can create a fear of failure, discouraging risk-taking and leading to frustration when setbacks occur. A growth mindset, on the other hand, shifts the focus to the learning process and personal growth rather than immediate outcomes.

Adopting this mentality can lead to greater resilience and success in all areas of life. It encourages men to embrace challenges, seek feedback, and persist even when things get tough. When you adopt a growth mindset, you no longer see failure as a reflection of your worth, but as a stepping stone toward growth.

Practical Steps to Develop a Growth Mindset

1. Embrace Challenges

One of the key principles of a growth mindset is viewing challenges as opportunities for growth rather than threats. Instead of shying away from difficult situations, lean into them. Challenges help you learn new skills, expand your capabilities, and prove that you are capable of more than you initially believed.

For example, if you're struggling with emotional vulnerability, facing difficult conversations with loved ones or opening up about your feelings may feel intimidating. However, each time you engage in these conversations, you develop greater emotional intelligence and communication skills. The more you practice, the more confident and competent you become.

2. Reframe Failures as Learning Opportunities

Failure is an inevitable part of life, but how you interpret failure can make all the difference in your personal growth. People with a fixed mindset often see failure as a sign of inadequacy or personal defeat. In contrast, those with a growth mindset view failure as a valuable learning opportunity.

When you experience setbacks—whether in relationships, career, or personal goals—ask yourself, "What can I learn from this?" Reflect on the situation and identify areas where you can grow or improve. By shifting your focus to the lessons gained, failure becomes a stepping stone toward future success rather than a roadblock.

3. Celebrate Effort, Not Just Results

In a fixed mindset, success is often measured solely by outcomes: the promotion, the award, the achievement. While results matter, a growth mindset emphasizes effort and progress. Acknowledge and celebrate the hard work you put into your goals, regardless of whether the outcome is exactly what you wanted.

For instance, if you've been working on managing your mental health or improving your relationships, celebrate the progress you've made, even if you're not yet where you want to be. Recognizing and valuing effort reinforces the idea that personal growth is an ongoing process, and it helps to build confidence and motivation.

4. Seek Feedback and Learn from Others

In a growth mindset, feedback is a critical tool for self-improvement. Instead of fearing criticism or seeing it as an attack on your abilities, seek out constructive feedback from others. Whether it's in your personal or professional life, asking for feedback shows that you're open to growth and eager to improve.

For men, who are often conditioned to appear strong and self-reliant, seeking feedback can feel uncomfortable. However, recognizing that feedback helps you identify blind spots, sharpen your skills, and grow emotionally can transform how you interact with others. Learning from those around you—whether colleagues, friends, or mentors—enriches your experience and expands your perspective.

The Importance of Self-Compassion

While a growth mindset emphasizes effort and learning, self-compassion plays a crucial role in how you treat yourself during the process. Self-compassion involves being kind and understanding to yourself, especially when things don't go as planned. Instead of criticizing or shaming yourself for mistakes, self-compassion allows you to approach setbacks with patience and empathy.

For many men, the notion of self-compassion can be foreign. Society often teaches that strength comes from toughness and stoicism, leading men to internalize their emotions and harshly criticize themselves for perceived failures. However, self-compassion is not about letting yourself off the hook— it's about recognizing that you are human, capable of mistakes, and worthy of kindness, even during difficult times.

Practical Steps to Cultivate Self-Compassion

1. Practice Self-Kindness

Self-kindness means treating yourself with the same care and understanding that you would offer to a friend. When you encounter difficulties or fall short of your goals, resist the urge to be overly critical or judgmental. Instead, remind yourself that it's okay to make mistakes and that no one is perfect.

For example, if you struggle with anxiety or frustration in personal relationships, rather than berating yourself for not handling situations perfectly, offer yourself reassurance. You might say, "I'm doing my best, and it's okay to have moments of weakness. I'll learn from this and do better next time." Self-kindness fosters a more compassionate and patient inner dialogue, which supports emotional well-being.

2. Acknowledge Your Humanity

Part of self-compassion is acknowledging that everyone experiences challenges and setbacks. You're not alone in facing difficulties. By recognizing that your struggles are part of the shared human experience, you reduce feelings of isolation and self-blame.

For instance, if you've encountered stress at work or difficulties in personal relationships, remind yourself that everyone deals with similar challenges at some point. By acknowledging this shared reality, you can let go of perfectionism and accept that growth takes time.

3. Practice Mindfulness

Mindfulness is the practice of being present in the moment without judgment. It involves acknowledging your thoughts and emotions without letting them control you. When you experience negative emotions—such as frustration, sadness, or anger—mindfulness allows you to observe them without getting caught up in them.

By practicing mindfulness, you become more attuned to your emotional state and can approach your feelings with curiosity rather than judgment. For instance, if you're feeling overwhelmed, take a moment to pause and breathe. Notice the sensation without trying to push it away or label it as "bad." Mindfulness helps you respond to emotions in a more balanced and compassionate way.

4. Forgive Yourself for Past Mistakes

We all carry regrets and moments from the past where we wish we had acted differently. Holding onto self-blame for past mistakes can prevent you from moving forward. Self-compassion involves forgiving yourself for past errors and recognizing that you did the best you could with the knowledge and resources you had at the time.

Forgiveness doesn't mean dismissing or excusing harmful behavior, but it does mean allowing yourself to let go of guilt and learn from the experience. When you forgive yourself, you create space for healing and growth.

The Benefits of Cultivating Growth and Self-Compassion

Cultivating a mindset of growth and self-compassion offers numerous benefits for personal development and emotional well-being. These practices allow you to:

- Increase Resilience: A growth mindset helps you navigate challenges with confidence, while self-compassion supports emotional recovery when things don't go as planned.
- Enhance Relationships: Emotional intelligence and empathy are nurtured by self-compassion, making you more patient and understanding in your interactions with others.
- Reduce Stress and Anxiety: By treating yourself with kindness and recognizing that growth is a gradual process, you reduce the pressure to be perfect, alleviating stress and anxiety.
- Promote Long-Term Success: A growth mindset encourages persistence and effort, which leads to greater personal and professional success over time.

In conclusion, cultivating a mindset of growth and self-compassion is foundational for empowered masculinity. By embracing challenges, treating yourself with kindness, and committing to personal growth, you develop emotional strength and resilience that support long-term well-being.

MASTERING RELATIONSHIPS:
COMMUNICATION, INTIMACY, AND PARTNERSHIP

For many men, the ability to form deep, meaningful connections can be hindered by societal expectations, emotional barriers, and misconceptions about masculinity. One of the key components to breaking through these obstacles is honest communication, which serves as the foundation for healthy, long-lasting relationships. Let's explore how communication, intimacy, and partnership work together to create stronger connections, and how men can learn to balance strength with vulnerability.

The Role of Honest Communication in Building Healthy Relationships

At the heart of every healthy relationship lies communication. Honest, open dialogue is not just about talking, but truly connecting with someone on a deeper level. For men, this can often be a challenge due to cultural conditioning that emphasizes stoicism and emotional restraint. However, understanding that vulnerability is a strength can be transformative in building strong, meaningful bonds.

Why Communication Is Vital:

Communication allows partners to express their needs, desires, and boundaries. It fosters trust, emotional intimacy, and mutual respect. In romantic relationships, open communication is the foundation upon which couples navigate life's complexities. Without it, misunderstandings, resentment, and distance can grow, weakening the relationship over time.

Honest communication involves being upfront about your thoughts, feelings, and concerns while also being receptive to the other person's perspective. It requires active listening, empathy, and a willingness to share even the more uncomfortable emotions.

Breaking Down Emotional Barriers:

Men often face internal barriers to honest communication, stemming from societal pressures to be emotionally stoic or "tough." These pressures can prevent men from expressing vulnerability, leading to misunderstandings in their relationships. However, when men recognize that sharing their emotions does not make them weak but rather strengthens their relationships, they begin to break free from these limiting beliefs.

Honest communication requires courage, particularly when it comes to expressing difficult emotions such as fear, sadness, or frustration. Yet, it's through these difficult conversations that deeper connections are forged. When men take the step to share their true selves with their partners, they create a space for intimacy and growth.

Intimacy: More Than Just Physical

Intimacy in relationships is often misunderstood, with many assuming it refers solely to physical closeness. However, true intimacy extends beyond the physical—it's about emotional, intellectual, and spiritual connection. Intimacy is cultivated through shared experiences, mutual understanding, and, importantly, communication.

Emotional Intimacy:

Emotional intimacy is the closeness that comes from being able to share one's innermost thoughts and feelings without fear of judgment. It's about being truly seen and understood by another person. For men, developing emotional intimacy can be a powerful experience, as it allows them to drop the armor they often wear and connect on a deeper level with their partners.

Building emotional intimacy requires time, trust, and a safe environment. It's fostered when both partners feel comfortable being vulnerable, knowing that their emotions will be met with empathy and respect. In this sense, emotional intimacy is a two-way street—it involves both the willingness to share and the ability to listen and understand.

Intellectual and Spiritual Intimacy:

Intellectual intimacy involves engaging in meaningful conversations, discussing ideas, and sharing perspectives on various aspects of life. It's about respecting each other's viewpoints and being open to learning from one another. For many couples, intellectual connection is just as important as emotional or physical closeness, as it provides a space for mental stimulation and growth.

Spiritual intimacy, on the other hand, refers to the sense of connection that comes from shared beliefs, values, or practices. This could involve shared religious beliefs, a commitment to personal growth, or a mutual desire to lead a life of purpose. Spiritual intimacy strengthens the bond between partners by aligning them on a deeper, more existential level.

Balancing Sensitivity and Strength in Romantic Partnerships

One of the great challenges many men face in relationships is finding the balance between sensitivity and strength. Traditional notions of masculinity often emphasize strength at the expense of sensitivity, leading men to suppress their emotions and vulnerability. However, true strength lies in being able to balance both—being emotionally available while also being resilient in the face of challenges.

The Strength in Sensitivity:

Sensitivity is often viewed as a feminine trait, yet it is essential for successful relationships. Being sensitive means being attuned to your partner's needs, emotions, and unspoken cues. It involves practicing empathy—understanding and sharing in the emotional experiences of others. Sensitivity allows men to respond to their partner's emotional needs with care and understanding, which fosters trust and closeness.

Men who embrace their sensitive side often find that their relationships become more harmonious and fulfilling. Rather than seeing sensitivity as a weakness, they recognize it as a strength that enhances their ability to connect with others on a deeper level. Sensitivity doesn't detract from strength—it complements it, allowing men to be emotionally available while maintaining their resolve and stability.

The Strength in Resilience:

On the flip side, strength in relationships is about resilience—having the ability to navigate difficult times without losing sight of the relationship's foundation. Strength in this context doesn't mean suppressing emotions or being stoic; it's about facing challenges head-on, communicating openly about difficulties, and working together to find solutions.

Resilience in relationships is about the long game—staying committed even when things get tough, being willing to compromise, and maintaining trust and support for one another through life's ups and downs. A strong relationship isn't one without challenges; it's one that can weather those challenges and come out stronger on the other side.

Nurturing Intimacy While Maintaining Personal Boundaries

While building intimacy is essential for a strong relationship, it's equally important to maintain personal boundaries. Boundaries ensure that both partners maintain their individuality and personal space within the relationship, preventing codependency or emotional burnout.

Respecting Personal Space:

In any relationship, there's a delicate balance between togetherness and individuality. While intimacy brings partners closer, personal boundaries protect each person's sense of self. Respecting personal space—both physical and emotional—is crucial for maintaining a healthy dynamic.

Healthy boundaries allow each partner to pursue their interests, spend time alone, and reflect on their needs without feeling smothered or obligated. When personal boundaries are respected, partners feel more secure, knowing that their individuality is valued within the relationship.

Communicating Boundaries:

Communicating personal boundaries openly is essential. Partners need to express their boundaries clearly and respectfully, whether they involve time, personal interests, emotional needs, or physical space. For example, one partner may need time alone to recharge, while the other may need regular emotional check-ins to feel secure. When both partners communicate their needs openly, they create a dynamic where both feel heard and respected.

Boundaries are not barriers—they are guidelines that help protect emotional and mental well-being. When boundaries are communicated and respected, they actually strengthen the bond between partners by fostering trust, respect, and understanding.

In mastering relationships, men must learn to embrace vulnerability, practice honest communication, and balance sensitivity with strength. Intimacy and partnership are strengthened when both partners feel seen, heard, and respected. By fostering open dialogue, respecting boundaries, and nurturing emotional intimacy, men can build relationships that are not only fulfilling but also resilient and enduring.

BALANCING SENSITIVITY AND STRENGTH IN ROMANTIC PARTNERSHIPS

In romantic relationships, the balance between sensitivity and strength is often a delicate and complex dynamic.

Society frequently presents these two qualities as opposing forces—strength is often associated with stoicism, control, and toughness, while sensitivity is linked to vulnerability, emotional openness, and care. For many men, navigating between these two poles can feel challenging, as they may struggle to reconcile the need to be strong with the importance of being emotionally available. However, true harmony in romantic partnerships comes when sensitivity and strength are seen not as contradictions but as complementary qualities that, when balanced, lead to deeper, more fulfilling relationships.

Understanding the True Nature of Strength

Before exploring how sensitivity can enhance strength, it's crucial to redefine what strength truly means in the context of relationships. Traditional views of strength often emphasize physical power, control, and the ability to face challenges without showing vulnerability. While these aspects of strength may have their place in certain situations, they are limited and often lead to emotional suppression or relational distance.

Strength in a romantic relationship is not about dominating or suppressing emotions but about resilience, emotional stability, and the ability to face challenges with a clear mind. It's about staying grounded during difficult times, supporting your partner when they need it most, and showing up consistently with reliability. Strength involves not only the capacity to face external challenges but also the courage to confront inner emotional struggles.

In relationships, strength means having the ability to:

- Hold space for your partner's emotions without feeling overwhelmed.
- Offer support when your partner is going through a tough time, while also maintaining your own emotional balance.
- Be vulnerable and honest about your own fears, challenges, and insecurities, without letting them dictate the course of the relationship.

A strong partner doesn't shy away from vulnerability. Instead, they recognize that true strength involves the courage to face emotional truths, both their own and their partner's.

Sensitivity: The Key to Emotional Connection

While strength ensures that a relationship can weather storms, sensitivity creates the emotional depth and connection that allow it to thrive. Sensitivity involves being attuned to your partner's emotional needs, being empathetic, and showing care and understanding in moments of vulnerability. For many men, sensitivity can feel like an uncomfortable space to inhabit, especially when societal messages equate emotional openness with weakness. However, in reality, sensitivity is one of the most powerful tools a man can bring to a relationship.

Being sensitive means paying attention to both verbal and non-verbal cues from your partner, listening with empathy, and responding in a way that honors their feelings. It also involves being aware of your own emotional state and understanding how it impacts your relationship.

Benefits of Sensitivity in Romantic Partnerships:

- Deepening emotional intimacy: Sensitivity allows for a deeper emotional connection between partners. When one person feels truly understood and supported, trust is built, and intimacy flourishes.
- Resolving conflicts with compassion: Sensitivity helps de-escalate arguments and resolve conflicts more effectively. When both partners approach disagreements with empathy, they are more likely to reach a resolution that strengthens the relationship rather than damages it.
- Strengthening communication: Being sensitive to your partner's needs helps create a safe space for honest communication, where both people feel free to express themselves without fear of judgment or rejection.

Sensitivity in relationships is not about being overly emotional or losing oneself in the emotions of the moment. Rather, it's about being present with your partner's emotional experience and responding in a way that fosters connection and healing.

How Sensitivity and Strength Complement Each Other

While sensitivity and strength may seem like opposing qualities, they are, in fact, complementary. A strong relationship requires both the stability that comes from strength and the emotional depth that sensitivity provides. When men embrace both qualities, they can create partnerships that are balanced, supportive, and resilient.

Here's how sensitivity and strength work together in romantic partnerships:

1. Supporting Through Difficult Times

When challenges arise in a relationship, strength ensures that both partners can face adversity with resilience and determination. However, without sensitivity, strength can come off as emotionally distant or unfeeling. Sensitivity ensures that strength is not cold or detached, but rather guided by empathy and care. By combining both, men can offer unwavering support while also being emotionally available, which strengthens the relationship during difficult times.

2. Building Emotional Safety

Emotional safety is key to a thriving relationship. While strength provides stability, it's sensitivity that creates the sense of safety and understanding that partners need to feel secure. A partner who is both strong and sensitive can create an environment where their partner feels safe to express their true selves without fear of being judged or dismissed. This emotional safety fosters intimacy and connection, which leads to a more fulfilling partnership.

3. Balancing Independence and Connection

Strength helps maintain healthy boundaries and independence within a relationship, ensuring that both partners have space to pursue their individual goals and interests. Sensitivity, on the other hand, strengthens the emotional connection between partners. Together, they allow for a relationship where both partners feel connected and supported, while also maintaining a sense of individuality and independence.

4. Handling Vulnerability with Courage

Vulnerability can be difficult for anyone, especially for men who may have been taught to hide their emotions. Strength provides the courage to face vulnerability, while sensitivity helps navigate those moments with care. When a man can show strength by embracing his vulnerability and express it with sensitivity, it creates an environment where emotional honesty is valued and where both partners can grow together.

Practical Tips for Balancing Sensitivity and Strength

Finding the balance between sensitivity and strength is a process that requires self-awareness, intentionality, and practice. Here are a few ways men can work towards achieving this balance in their romantic relationships:

- Practice active listening: One of the best ways to show sensitivity is to truly listen to your partner without interrupting or offering solutions. Allow your partner to express themselves fully, and respond with empathy and understanding.
- Be honest about your emotions: Strength involves being vulnerable enough to share your own emotions. Whether you're feeling stressed, upset, or unsure, communicating openly with your partner builds trust and intimacy.
- Set healthy boundaries: Strength isn't just about protecting your partner—it's also about maintaining your own well-being. Set clear boundaries that protect your time, energy, and emotional space, while also respecting your partner's needs.
- Check in with yourself regularly: Balancing sensitivity and strength requires self-awareness. Regularly reflect on

your emotional state, your relationship dynamics, and whether you're maintaining a healthy balance between being emotionally available and resilient.

- Show compassion in difficult moments: Whether your partner is going through a tough time or you're dealing with a conflict, lead with sensitivity and compassion. Offer support, but also remain grounded and strong enough to handle the situation without being overwhelmed.

In romantic partnerships, the balance between sensitivity and strength creates a foundation for deep, meaningful connection. By embracing both qualities, men can foster relationships that are not only emotionally fulfilling but also resilient and enduring. Sensitivity allows men to connect with their partners on a deeper emotional level, while strength provides the stability and courage to face challenges together. When combined, these two qualities create a powerful dynamic that leads to healthier, happier, and more connected partnerships.

BALANCING CAREER,
FAMILY, AND PERSONAL GROWTH

Men may find themselves juggling the demands of career aspirations, family responsibilities, and their own personal growth. Striking the right balance between these three aspects of life is essential not only for personal well-being but also for nurturing relationships and achieving long-term success. Balancing career, family, and personal growth is not just about time management; it's about aligning your values and priorities to create a fulfilling, meaningful life.

The Importance of Balance

The first step toward achieving balance between career, family, and personal growth is recognizing why it's necessary. Men are often socialized to prioritize their careers above all else, equating professional success with self-worth and personal fulfillment. However, when work dominates every aspect of life, it can lead to burnout, strained relationships, and a loss of personal identity. True fulfillment comes when you cultivate a harmonious balance that allows you to thrive both professionally and personally.

By finding balance, you:

- Prevent burnout: Overworking leads to physical and emotional exhaustion. Balance allows you to maintain high performance without sacrificing your mental health.
- Strengthen relationships: Quality time spent with family and loved ones builds stronger connections, which leads to emotional fulfillment.

- Promote personal growth: Investing time in self-improvement, hobbies, and personal development ensures that you continue evolving as an individual, outside of your career and family roles.

Setting Priorities: Clarifying What Matters Most

To create balance, the first step is to set clear priorities. This requires reflection on what matters most to you and how you want to distribute your time and energy. For many men, the struggle comes from feeling pulled in different directions—between career demands, family obligations, and the desire for personal time. The key is to identify your core values and align your daily actions with those values.

Ask yourself:

- What are my long-term goals for my career, family, and personal life?
- Am I sacrificing one area of my life for another? If so, why?
- What brings me the greatest sense of fulfillment, and how can I incorporate more of that into my daily routine?

When you're clear on your priorities, it becomes easier to make decisions that support your overall well-being. For example, if family time is a top priority, you'll be more intentional about setting boundaries at work to protect that time. If personal growth is important, you'll carve out time for self-reflection, hobbies, or learning new skills.

Time Management: Creating Structure Without Sacrifice

Once you've set your priorities, the next step is to manage your time effectively. Many men struggle to balance their professional ambitions with family and personal life because they don't have a clear system for managing their time. Time management isn't about rigid schedules or sacrificing one area of life for another; it's about creating structure that allows you to be fully present in each aspect of your life.

Here are some strategies to help you manage your time effectively:

1. Time blocking: This involves scheduling specific blocks of time for different areas of your life. For example, you might dedicate mornings to work tasks, afternoons to family time, and evenings to personal growth or hobbies. Time blocking ensures that each area of your life gets the attention it deserves without feeling scattered or overwhelmed.

2. Setting boundaries: Establishing boundaries is essential for maintaining balance. This means setting limits on work hours, saying no to unnecessary commitments, and protecting your personal and family time. For example, you might set a rule that you don't check work emails after a certain time, or you dedicate weekends solely to family activities.

3. Delegation and outsourcing: You don't have to do everything yourself. In both your professional and personal life, delegating tasks to others can free up time for the things that matter most. At work, delegate tasks to team members when appropriate, and at home, consider outsourcing tasks like cleaning or meal prep to create more time for family and personal pursuits.

4. Prioritizing self-care: Many men neglect self-care in the pursuit of career success or family obligations, but personal well-being is the foundation of balance. Make time for activities that recharge you, whether that's exercise, meditation, reading, or spending time outdoors. When you're physically and emotionally well, you're better equipped to handle the demands of work and family life.

Balancing Career and Family: Nurturing Both Roles

For many men, the most challenging part of achieving balance is finding harmony between career and family life. Often, professional success is viewed as a key marker of masculinity, leading men to prioritize work at the expense of family relationships. However, neglecting family time can have long-term negative effects on your relationships and emotional well-being.

The key to balancing career and family is intentionality. This means being present and engaged in both areas of your life, rather than allowing one to dominate the other. Here's how to approach it:

- Be present with family: When you're spending time with your family, be fully present. Put away your phone, close your laptop, and engage with your loved ones. Quality family time isn't just about being physically present; it's about actively participating in your relationships and making meaningful connections.
- Set work boundaries: Establish clear boundaries around work hours, especially if you work from home. Communicate these boundaries with your employer and

your family, so everyone is on the same page. For example, you might set a rule that you don't take work calls during family dinners or that weekends are reserved for family activities.

- Involve your family in career decisions: When making major career decisions, such as accepting a promotion or taking on a new project, consider how it will impact your family life. Involve your partner and family in these decisions, so they feel included and supported.
- Plan family time: Just as you schedule work meetings, make sure to schedule family time. Whether it's weekly family dinners, weekend outings, or vacations, planning family time ensures that it doesn't get overshadowed by work responsibilities.

Personal Growth: Making Time for Yourself

While career and family are important, personal growth should not be neglected. Many men put their own needs on the back burner in the pursuit of success or the desire to provide for their family. However, personal growth is essential for long-term fulfillment and well-being.

Personal growth involves continuously evolving as an individual—mentally, emotionally, and spiritually. It's about cultivating your passions, learning new skills, and taking time for self-reflection. Here's how to make time for personal growth while balancing career and family:

- Schedule personal time: Just as you schedule work tasks and family time, make sure to schedule time for yourself. This could be early morning before work, during lunch breaks, or in the evenings after family time. Use this time for activities that nourish your soul, whether that's reading, journaling, practicing a hobby, or working on a personal project.

- Pursue lifelong learning: Personal growth often comes through learning new things. This could involve taking a class, attending workshops, or simply reading books on topics that interest you. Continuously expanding your knowledge and skills not only enhances your personal growth but also benefits your career and relationships.
- Reflect on your values and goals: Regularly take time to reflect on your personal values and goals. Are you living in alignment with your core beliefs? Are you pursuing goals that bring you true fulfillment? Self-reflection is a powerful tool for personal growth, helping you stay on course and make necessary adjustments when needed.
- Find a mentor or coach: Personal growth is often accelerated when you have guidance from someone who has walked the path before you. Consider finding a mentor or coach who can help you navigate challenges, offer advice, and hold you accountable for your personal and professional development.

Achieving Balance: The Ongoing Process

Balancing career, family, and personal growth is not a one-time achievement—it's an ongoing process that requires constant evaluation and adjustment. Life is dynamic, and what works for you at one stage may need to be recalibrated as circumstances change. The key is to remain flexible and open to making changes when necessary.

Evaluate your balance regularly: Periodically reflect on how well you're balancing the different areas of your life. Are you feeling fulfilled and energized, or are you experiencing burnout and stress? Are your relationships thriving, or are they suffering due to work demands? By regularly evaluating your balance, you can make adjustments as needed to ensure that you're living a life that aligns with your values and goals.

TRATEGIES FOR BEING AN ENGAGED FATHER AND PARTNER

The role of fathers and partners has evolved significantly, moving away from the traditional model of distant providers to more engaged, emotionally available, and active participants in family life. Being an engaged father and partner not only strengthens family bonds but also positively impacts children's development, relationship satisfaction, and personal well-being. However, balancing the responsibilities of fatherhood and partnership with the demands of work and personal growth can be challenging.

Here are some key strategies for being an engaged and present father and partner:

1. Prioritize Quality Time with Family

One of the most impactful ways to be an engaged father and partner is by prioritizing quality time with your family. This means being fully present and actively involved during family interactions, whether it's spending time with your children or deepening your connection with your partner.

- Scheduled family time: In a busy world, family time can easily be overshadowed by work obligations and daily distractions. Make a conscious effort to schedule regular family activities, such as weekly family dinners, outings, or game nights. These moments provide opportunities for bonding and creating shared memories.

- Be present: Quality time is not just about being physically present but also emotionally engaged. Put away distractions like your phone or laptop during family time. Focus on listening, engaging in conversations, and being mindful of what's happening with your children and partner. Active presence helps build trust and deepens relationships.

- Create traditions: Family traditions—whether they're holiday rituals, weekend activities, or special family projects—create a sense of unity and stability. They can be as simple as a Sunday breakfast or as elaborate as an annual vacation, but they should involve everyone's participation and foster a strong family connection.

2. Practice Open and Honest Communication

Open communication is a cornerstone of any strong relationship, especially when it comes to parenting and partnerships. Effective communication fosters trust, helps resolve conflicts, and ensures that everyone feels heard and valued.

- Create a safe space for expression: Encourage your children and partner to express their thoughts, feelings, and concerns openly without fear of judgment. This creates a supportive environment where family members feel comfortable sharing what's on their minds, whether it's about school, work, or personal issues.

- Model emotional intelligence: As an engaged father and partner, it's important to model emotional intelligence by expressing your own feelings in a healthy way. Let your family see that it's okay to be vulnerable, to admit when you're feeling stressed, or to ask for help when needed. This not only strengthens your relationship but also teaches children emotional regulation.

- Be an active listener: Engage in conversations with full attention, showing that you genuinely care about what your children or partner are saying. Ask questions, offer empathy, and avoid interrupting or offering solutions too quickly. Sometimes, simply listening is the most important thing you can do.

3. Show Affection and Appreciation

Expressing love and appreciation for your family is crucial to creating a nurturing and supportive environment. Acts of affection, whether verbal or physical, help maintain emotional closeness and build strong relationships.

- Regularly express love: Tell your partner and children that you love them regularly. Verbal affirmations of love and appreciation, especially when specific and sincere, foster emotional connection. Compliment your partner's efforts or let your child know how proud you are of their achievements.

- Physical affection: Physical touch is a powerful way to communicate care and affection. Whether it's a hug, a kiss, or simply holding hands, these small gestures of physical connection build emotional intimacy. Engaged fathers often make a point of hugging their children, playing with them, or simply sitting close while watching a movie.

- Celebrate achievements and milestones: Make a habit of celebrating the small and big victories in your family's life. Whether it's a promotion at work, a school achievement, or a personal milestone, recognition helps family members feel valued and supported.

4. Be a Role Model

As a father and partner, you have the opportunity to model the behaviors and values you want to instill in your children and bring into your relationship. Children, in particular, learn by example, and the way you treat others, manage responsibilities, and face challenges will shape their understanding of these dynamics.

- Model respect and empathy: Show respect for your partner and others in your life, both in words and actions. Children observe and learn from how you treat their mother or other significant people, and this shapes their perception of healthy relationships.

- Demonstrate work-life balance: Teach your children the importance of balancing work and family life by setting clear boundaries between the two. When you actively take time for family while managing professional responsibilities, you model the value of prioritizing what truly matters.

- Show resilience in the face of challenges: Life will inevitably bring challenges, and how you handle these situations as a father and partner sets an example for your family. Show resilience, perseverance, and the ability to ask for help when needed. Encourage problem-solving, teamwork, and a positive attitude in the face of adversity.

5. Involve Yourself in Parenting Tasks

Being an engaged father means actively participating in parenting tasks, both big and small. Whether it's helping with schoolwork, attending parent-teacher conferences, or simply making dinner, involvement in day-to-day parenting creates a strong bond between you and your children.

- Be hands-on with daily tasks: From diaper changes to helping with homework or driving the kids to extracurricular activities, being hands-on in daily parenting routines helps you stay connected to your children's lives. It also models to your children that fatherhood involves more than just providing financially; it's about emotional and practical support.

- Support your partner: Parenting is a shared responsibility, and being an engaged father also means supporting your partner in co-parenting duties. This fosters a sense of teamwork and equality in the relationship. Offering to take on household or childcare tasks when your partner is overwhelmed demonstrates your commitment to the family's well-being.

- Teach and guide: Beyond practical tasks, an engaged father is also an active teacher and guide. Use everyday situations as teaching moments to pass on life skills, values, and knowledge. Whether it's teaching your child how to handle conflict, manage money, or navigate relationships, these lessons will leave a lasting impact.

6. Be Involved in Your Partner's Life

While being an engaged father is crucial, being a present and supportive partner is equally important. Nurturing your romantic relationship will not only strengthen the bond between you and your partner but will also create a stable, loving environment for your children.

- Stay connected emotionally: In the busyness of life, it's easy for partners to drift apart emotionally. Make time to reconnect with your partner regularly through deep conversations, shared activities, or even date nights. Show interest in your partner's life, dreams, and challenges, and provide emotional support when needed.

- Share responsibilities equally: A strong partnership involves sharing both the mental and physical load of household and parenting tasks. Support your partner by taking on equal responsibilities, ensuring that neither partner feels burdened or overwhelmed.

- Keep the romance alive: While the demands of parenting and work may make it difficult to prioritize romance, small gestures can go a long way in maintaining intimacy. Surprise your partner with thoughtful acts, express appreciation, and make time for each other outside of the parental role.

7. Maintain Personal Growth Alongside Family Responsibilities

Lastly, as much as being an engaged father and partner is important, so too is your own personal growth and well-being. You cannot pour from an empty cup, and taking time for self-care ensures you are emotionally and mentally prepared to give your best to your family.

- Pursue personal hobbies and interests: Engaged fathers and partners are also well-rounded individuals who continue to nurture their passions and hobbies. Carving out time for activities that recharge and inspire you not only benefits your mental health but also sets an example for your children about the importance of pursuing passions.

- Maintain friendships and social support: Having a strong social network outside of the family unit is essential for personal well-being. Engaged fathers maintain friendships, participate in social activities, and seek out community support when needed. This external support system helps relieve the pressure on family dynamics and keeps you emotionally grounded.

- Seek personal development: Personal growth and self-improvement should continue even after becoming a father and partner. Whether through reading, learning new skills, or engaging in personal reflection, keep growing as an individual. A strong, self-aware man contributes positively to his relationships and serves as a role model for his children.

SPIRITUALITY AND MASCULINITY

Masculinity is often discussed in terms of external success, achievements, strength, and power. However, there is another dimension that shapes an empowered form of masculinity—spirituality. Spirituality provides a deeper connection to purpose, offering men a sense of meaning and guiding principles that go beyond material success or societal expectations.

Spirituality plays a crucial role in helping men navigate life's challenges, fostering emotional resilience, and nurturing a strong sense of identity that is grounded in internal values rather than external pressures. By tapping into a higher purpose, men can cultivate a more holistic, empowered masculinity that integrates sensitivity, strength, compassion, and wisdom.

Let's explore how spirituality can shape and transform masculinity:

1. Spirituality as a Foundation for Inner Strength

Many traditional models of masculinity emphasize physical strength, toughness, and stoicism. While these traits can be valuable, they often come at the expense of emotional and mental well-being. Spirituality, on the other hand, encourages the development of inner strength—rooted in self-awareness, emotional intelligence, and a connection to something greater than oneself.

Developing inner resilience: Spirituality encourages men to cultivate an inner fortitude that helps them withstand adversity. Rather than relying solely on external displays of toughness, spiritually grounded men develop resilience through practices like mindfulness, meditation, and prayer. This inner resilience allows men to face life's difficulties with grace and composure, without the need to suppress emotions or maintain a façade of invulnerability.

A source of guidance in times of crisis: When life becomes challenging, spiritual beliefs and practices offer a sense of purpose and direction. Whether it's through religious faith, meditation, or a connection to nature, spirituality provides men with a way to reflect on life's deeper questions and find meaning even in difficult circumstances. This higher perspective allows men to navigate crises with a sense of hope and trust in something greater than the immediate situation.

Embracing humility: Spirituality fosters humility, helping men recognize their limitations and acknowledge that they don't have all the answers. Rather than viewing vulnerability as a weakness, spiritually empowered men understand that it is through accepting their vulnerability and seeking wisdom from a higher source that true strength is found. This humility helps men shed the societal expectation of having to "be strong all the time" and instead embrace the deeper strength that comes from aligning with a higher purpose.

2. Connecting to a Higher Purpose

One of the most significant benefits of spirituality is the sense of higher purpose it brings to life. In a world driven by materialism and the pursuit of external success, many men find themselves feeling lost, disconnected, or unfulfilled. Spirituality offers a path to discovering and aligning with a deeper purpose that transcends societal pressures or personal ambition.

The search for meaning: Spirituality encourages men to ask questions about the meaning of life, their role in the world, and the legacy they want to leave behind. These reflections often lead to a greater understanding of purpose, which can be the driving force behind a man's decisions, actions, and relationships. Having a strong sense of purpose allows men to live with intention and integrity, making choices that align with their deepest values.

Beyond material success: While traditional notions of masculinity often focus on achievements like wealth, power, and status, spirituality invites men to redefine success in terms of personal growth, service to others, and living in alignment with their values. Men who connect with a higher purpose understand that true fulfillment comes not from external accolades, but from living a life of meaning and contribution.

Serving others: Many spiritual traditions emphasize the importance of service, compassion, and helping those in need. Spirituality encourages men to use their strengths and abilities for the benefit of others, whether through acts of kindness, mentorship, or community involvement. By serving a higher purpose, men can move beyond the self-centered pursuit of success and instead focus on creating positive change in the world.

3. Integrating Spiritual Practices into Daily Life

Spirituality is not just an abstract concept but can be woven into the fabric of daily life. By incorporating spiritual practices into everyday routines, men can maintain a sense of connection to their higher purpose and cultivate qualities like patience, compassion, and mindfulness.

Mindfulness and meditation: One of the most accessible ways to integrate spirituality into daily life is through mindfulness or meditation practices. These practices help men stay present, reduce stress, and develop a deeper connection to their inner selves. Regular meditation can also enhance emotional regulation, making it easier to navigate the ups and downs of life with a calm and centered mindset.

Journaling and reflection: Keeping a journal is a powerful tool for spiritual growth. Men can use journaling as a way to reflect on their thoughts, emotions, and experiences, and to explore deeper questions about their purpose and values. Writing down insights or lessons learned from challenging situations can help clarify one's path and align actions with a higher purpose.

Rituals and traditions: Many spiritual practices involve rituals or traditions that help anchor individuals in their beliefs. Whether it's attending religious services, engaging in personal rituals like lighting candles or reciting affirmations, or simply spending time in nature, these practices create a sense of sacredness and connection to something larger than oneself.

4. The Role of Spirituality in Emotional Healing

Spirituality also plays a crucial role in emotional healing, helping men process pain, trauma, and unresolved emotions. Through spiritual practices, men can find the space to acknowledge and release difficult feelings, ultimately leading to greater emotional freedom and peace.

Healing from past wounds: Many men carry unresolved emotional wounds from childhood, relationships, or life experiences. Spirituality offers a path to healing by providing tools for forgiveness, acceptance, and letting go. Whether through prayer, meditation, or rituals, spirituality can help men release old patterns of pain and open themselves to new possibilities for emotional growth and healing.

Cultivating self-compassion: Spirituality encourages men to develop self-compassion, allowing them to treat themselves with kindness and understanding, even when they fall short of their own expectations. This is especially important in a society that often teaches men to be hard on themselves or to suppress their emotions. Self-compassion nurtures emotional well-being and strengthens a man's ability to cope with life's challenges in a healthy way.

Finding peace in surrender: Many spiritual teachings emphasize the importance of surrender—letting go of the need to control everything and trusting in a higher power or the flow of life. For men who have been taught to be in control at all times, this can be a transformative shift. Surrendering to life's uncertainties and trusting in a higher purpose allows men to experience greater peace, reducing anxiety and stress.

5. Spirituality and Masculinity in Relationships

Spirituality can have a profound impact on relationships, whether it's with a partner, family, or community. A spiritually grounded man approaches relationships with a sense of compassion, empathy, and understanding, prioritizing emotional connection and mutual growth.

Deepening emotional intimacy: Spirituality fosters deeper emotional intimacy in relationships by encouraging men to be more present, open, and vulnerable with their loved ones. Rather than focusing on dominance or control, spiritually empowered men seek to connect on a soul level, cultivating trust, empathy, and emotional safety in their relationships.

Nurturing spiritual growth together: In romantic partnerships, spirituality can be a shared journey that deepens the connection between partners. Engaging in spiritual practices together, such as meditation, prayer, or attending spiritual gatherings, can create a bond that goes beyond the physical or emotional aspects of the relationship. It allows both partners to grow together, supporting each other's personal and spiritual evolution.

Building a compassionate community: Spirituality also encourages men to build and nurture compassionate communities. By fostering relationships based on mutual respect, empathy, and service, men can create networks of support and connection that strengthen both their personal lives and the broader community.

6. Empowered Masculinity Through Spiritual Leadership

An often overlooked aspect of masculinity is the role of spiritual leadership. Spiritual leaders are not defined by their dominance or authority, but by their ability to inspire, guide, and serve others with humility and integrity. This type of leadership is deeply rooted in a man's connection to his higher purpose and values.

Leading with compassion and integrity: Spiritual leadership emphasizes leading with compassion, empathy, and a commitment to serving others. Men who embody spiritual leadership prioritize the well-being of those they lead, whether in their families, workplaces, or communities. This type of leadership is not about control or power but about empowering others to reach their full potential.

Inspiring others through example: One of the most powerful ways to lead spiritually is by example. Men who live in alignment with their spiritual values—such as honesty, kindness, and humility—naturally inspire others to do the same. By modeling these qualities, spiritually empowered men become leaders who positively influence the people around them.

Spirituality plays an essential role in shaping a more empowered, holistic form of masculinity. By connecting to a higher purpose, cultivating inner strength, and embracing spiritual practices, men can navigate life's challenges with greater resilience, compassion, and wisdom. Spirituality not only enhances personal growth but also deepens relationships, strengthens communities, and nurtures a sense of fulfillment that goes beyond material success. Empowered masculinity is not just about external strength— it's about aligning with a higher purpose and living a life of integrity, compassion, and service.

THE BENEFITS OF SPIRITUAL PRACTICES IN FOSTERING PEACE, CLARITY, AND DIRECTION

Spiritual practices are tools that can help men achieve a sense of peace, clarity, and direction in their lives. These practices, ranging from meditation to prayer, mindfulness to journaling, and even moments of solitude, offer profound psychological and emotional benefits. They provide a structure through which men can reflect on their lives, connect with their inner selves, and find answers to the deeper questions that define their purpose. In a world filled with external distractions and pressures, spiritual practices serve as a sanctuary for personal growth, introspection, and alignment with higher values.

Here's how spiritual practices can foster peace, clarity, and direction in a man's life:

1. Fostering Inner Peace

Spiritual practices are invaluable for cultivating a sense of inner peace. In today's fast-paced world, men are often bombarded with stress, responsibilities, and expectations that can lead to emotional turmoil, anxiety, or burnout. Engaging in spiritual practices helps men create an internal calm amidst external chaos.

- Reducing stress and anxiety: Meditation, mindfulness, and deep breathing exercises are powerful spiritual tools that help men regulate their nervous systems. These practices allow individuals to step away from the mental noise of daily life, quieting the mind and promoting relaxation. By focusing on the present moment and tuning out distractions, men can reduce anxiety and find peace within themselves.

- Emotional balance: Through spiritual practices, men can cultivate emotional balance and resilience. Meditation, prayer, and reflection can help men process emotions in a healthy way, allowing them to release negative feelings such as anger, frustration, or fear. Spiritual practices create the mental and emotional space necessary to find peace, even in the face of challenging situations.

- Connection to a higher purpose: Many spiritual practices encourage men to connect with something greater than themselves—a higher power, the universe, or the flow of life. This connection provides comfort, reducing the feeling of being overwhelmed by life's demands. Knowing that they are part of a larger purpose or plan allows men to feel more at ease and grounded, fostering a deep sense of inner peace.

2. Gaining Clarity in Life

Spiritual practices offer men a way to achieve clarity in their thoughts, emotions, and decisions. When life becomes overwhelming, spiritual tools like meditation, journaling, or silent reflection can help men clear mental fog, gain insight, and better understand their paths.

- Mental clarity through reflection: Journaling and meditation are two spiritual practices that can help men organize their thoughts and identify patterns in their thinking. Regular journaling allows men to release mental clutter by putting their thoughts and feelings into words. This process brings clarity to internal conflicts, allowing men to better understand their motivations, desires, and goals.

- Making better decisions: When faced with difficult decisions or uncertain circumstances, spiritual practices can guide men toward more thoughtful, intentional choices. Practices like meditation and prayer offer a pause, allowing men to connect with their intuition and reflect on their values. Instead of reacting impulsively, men can make decisions that are aligned with their purpose and long-term goals.

- Aligning with inner wisdom: Spiritual practices often bring men in touch with their inner wisdom—the intuitive voice that knows what's best for their growth and well-being. By slowing down and listening to this inner voice through practices like mindfulness or quiet reflection, men can gain clarity on the next steps they need to take in life. This clarity helps them move forward with confidence and conviction.

3. Finding Direction and Purpose

One of the most profound benefits of spiritual practices is their ability to provide men with a clear sense of direction and purpose. In a world where many men feel pressured to meet societal expectations or chase external achievements, spirituality offers a deeper, more meaningful way to discover their true path.

- Connecting to personal purpose: Spiritual practices allow men to explore the deeper questions of life: Why am I here? What is my purpose? What do I truly value? Practices like meditation, prayer, and contemplation encourage men to look beyond the surface of daily life and connect with their core values and desires. This self-exploration leads to a clearer understanding of their personal mission and the impact they want to make on the world.

- Overcoming external distractions: The modern world is full of distractions, from social media to work pressures to societal expectations. These distractions can pull men away from their true purpose and create a sense of confusion or dissatisfaction. Spiritual practices offer a way to cut through the noise and reconnect with what truly matters. By regularly engaging in meditation, journaling, or spiritual study, men can stay focused on their deeper purpose, avoiding the pull of superficial pursuits.

- Building a life of intentionality: When men engage in spiritual practices, they are more likely to live with intentionality. Rather than being swept along by the demands of others or the fast pace of modern life, men who practice spirituality take control of their time, energy, and focus. They make choices that are aligned with their higher purpose, leading to a more fulfilling and directed life.

4. Emotional Healing and Release

Many spiritual practices help men heal emotional wounds and release past trauma, clearing the way for greater peace and clarity in life. Without emotional healing, it can be difficult to find direction or connect to a higher purpose.

- Healing through meditation and mindfulness: Mindfulness practices allow men to sit with their emotions without judgment, creating a space for healing and release. By observing their thoughts and feelings from a place of detachment, men can process old pain, forgive themselves or others, and let go of emotional baggage that no longer serves them.

- The role of forgiveness in spiritual growth: Forgiveness is a key element in many spiritual traditions, and it can be a powerful tool for emotional healing. Spiritual practices like prayer, reflection, or journaling can help men forgive themselves for past mistakes or release resentment toward others. This process of forgiveness brings emotional freedom, clearing away negativity and making room for peace and clarity.

- Letting go of the need for control: Many spiritual practices emphasize surrender—letting go of the need to control every aspect of life and trusting in a higher power or the natural flow of events. This surrender brings immense relief from stress, anxiety, and overthinking. By embracing the uncertainty of life, men can find peace in knowing that they don't have to have all the answers or be in control of everything at all times.

5. Spiritual Practices That Foster Peace, Clarity, and Direction

There are numerous spiritual practices that men can incorporate into their daily lives to foster a greater sense of peace, clarity, and direction. Some of these practices include:

- Meditation: Sitting in silence and focusing on the breath or a mantra helps calm the mind, reduce stress, and bring clarity to thoughts. Meditation also enhances self-awareness, helping men better understand their emotions and desires.

- Mindfulness: Mindfulness is the practice of being fully present in the moment, without judgment or distraction. By staying mindful throughout the day, men can reduce anxiety, improve focus, and gain greater clarity in their decision-making.

- Journaling: Writing down thoughts, emotions, and reflections in a journal allows men to process their experiences and gain insight into their inner world. Journaling can help clarify goals, release pent-up emotions, and identify patterns in behavior or thinking.

- Prayer or contemplation: For those with a religious or spiritual faith, prayer can be a powerful way to connect with a higher power and seek guidance. Contemplation, whether through nature or quiet reflection, offers similar benefits, providing men with moments of introspection and clarity.

- Solitude and nature: Spending time in solitude or connecting with nature can offer a deep sense of peace and clarity. Nature, in particular, provides a calming environment where men can reflect on their lives, feel connected to something larger, and find direction in their thoughts.

HANDLING CRISIS:
THE MASCULINE APPROACH TO ADVERSITY

Life inevitably brings moments of crisis—whether personal, professional, or emotional. These challenging moments test a man's character, strength, and resilience. The way men face crises has traditionally been framed through the lens of stoicism, suppressing emotions, and simply "powering through." However, a more evolved masculine approach involves confronting adversity with both grace and strength. This balance enables men to not only endure difficulties but to grow from them.

In this chapter, we explore how to navigate crises using strategies that harness inner strength, emotional intelligence, and a growth mindset. Facing adversity with grace is not about denying the gravity of the situation but about approaching it with clarity, self-awareness, and the determination to emerge stronger.

Understanding Crisis: Defining Personal and Professional Adversity

A crisis can take many forms, from sudden job loss to a health scare, from the breakdown of a relationship to financial hardship. What defines a crisis is the disruption it causes to our sense of stability and security. It shakes the foundation on which we've built our lives, forcing us to reassess and recalibrate.

- Personal Crises: These include health challenges, family issues, relationship breakdowns, or emotional traumas.

Personal crises tend to hit the core of our identity, questioning our sense of worth, purpose, and well-being.

- Professional Crises: These can involve job loss, career setbacks, failure in business, or conflicts with colleagues or leadership. Professional crises often trigger feelings of inadequacy or failure, as men may tie much of their self-worth to their careers.

Regardless of the nature of the crisis, how men choose to respond to these challenges defines their growth. The goal is to learn how to face these moments with a balanced masculine approach that combines emotional awareness with determined action.

Harnessing Emotional Resilience

The first step to handling a crisis with grace is understanding and managing your emotions. Crises often evoke a wide range of powerful emotions—fear, anger, anxiety, or even shame. Many men are taught to suppress these feelings or hide them under a mask of strength. However, true resilience is about acknowledging emotions, processing them, and then using that emotional clarity to move forward.

- Acknowledge Your Emotions: Ignoring your feelings during a crisis can lead to long-term emotional harm, causing repressed anger or grief. Acknowledging that you feel scared, vulnerable, or upset is not a sign of weakness. It is a necessary step to processing the situation. By recognizing your emotions, you can address them in healthy ways—such as through conversation, journaling, or mindfulness.

- Emotional Regulation: Emotional intelligence plays a key role in crisis management. When faced with adversity, it is easy to allow emotions to overwhelm your decision-making process, leading to impulsive or irrational actions. Learning to regulate emotions through deep breathing, mindfulness practices, or simply stepping back for reflection helps you respond more thoughtfully to challenges. By keeping emotions in check, you gain the mental clarity needed to navigate the situation more effectively.

- Develop a Support System: One of the most overlooked yet essential aspects of emotional resilience is having a strong support system. In times of crisis, turning to trusted friends, family, or mentors for guidance and emotional support can make an enormous difference. Asking for help or leaning on others during tough times does not diminish your strength—it enhances it by allowing you to benefit from collective wisdom and care.

Taking Decisive Action in Times of Crisis

While emotional regulation is crucial, action is the key to emerging from a crisis. Inaction or avoidance can make a crisis worse, leading to deeper feelings of helplessness or despair. Therefore, a key aspect of handling adversity is taking decisive, well-considered action.

- Assess the Situation with Clarity: The first step in taking action is gaining a clear understanding of the crisis. What are the root causes? What are the immediate threats or risks? Often, crises can seem overwhelming because they are emotionally charged, but by breaking down the situation into manageable parts, you can more easily see what needs to be done. A calm, objective assessment is critical to making informed decisions.

- Create a Plan of Action: Once you have assessed the situation, develop a practical and strategic plan for how to proceed. This plan doesn't have to solve every aspect of the crisis but should focus on immediate steps that can stabilize the situation. Having a plan, even a simple one, provides a sense of control and direction, reducing feelings of chaos or overwhelm.

- Embrace Adaptability: In a crisis, plans may not always unfold as expected, so being adaptable is crucial. The masculine ideal of unyielding strength can sometimes be counterproductive in these moments. True strength lies in the ability to pivot, adjust, and find alternative solutions when necessary. Rather than rigidly sticking to one course of action, embrace a mindset of flexibility, allowing you to respond to new developments with agility.

Building Mental Toughness

Mental toughness is an essential component of handling crises with strength. It's about cultivating the perseverance and grit needed to push through difficult times without giving up. Mental toughness doesn't mean suppressing emotions or ignoring hardship; rather, it's about building the capacity to endure challenges while maintaining focus and determination.

- Perseverance and Patience: One of the hallmarks of mental toughness is the ability to persevere through extended periods of difficulty. Many crises cannot be resolved overnight. Whether it's rebuilding after a financial loss or healing from a personal trauma, the process takes time. Learning to be patient, while continuing to take small, consistent steps toward resolution, is key to emerging from adversity stronger.

- Developing a Growth Mindset: Viewing crises as opportunities for growth rather than purely negative experiences builds mental resilience. A growth mindset allows you to see failure, setbacks, or adversity as necessary steps in your journey toward personal development. Every challenge becomes a lesson—a chance to learn something new about yourself, your strengths, and areas for improvement.

- Self-Discipline and Focus: During a crisis, it's easy to become distracted or lose motivation. Self-discipline is essential for staying focused on your goals and pushing through the temptation to give up. Establishing routines, sticking to healthy habits, and setting daily objectives can provide a sense of structure and normalcy even when life feels chaotic.

Embracing Vulnerability: The Gateway to Strength

A key part of handling adversity with grace is embracing vulnerability. Many men see vulnerability as a weakness— something to be hidden or avoided. But vulnerability is a powerful source of strength when approached with courage and self-awareness.

- Admitting Uncertainty: During a crisis, it's okay to admit that you don't have all the answers. No one does. Acknowledging that you are uncertain or struggling allows you to open yourself to new perspectives, seek guidance, and approach the situation with humility. Admitting vulnerability in moments of crisis fosters deeper connections with others who can offer help, wisdom, or support.

- Letting Go of Perfectionism: Perfectionism can be a major obstacle during a crisis, as it creates unrealistic expectations and increases pressure. Instead of striving to handle the crisis flawlessly, allow yourself to make mistakes and learn from them. Letting go of perfectionism enables you to approach the situation with more flexibility and reduces feelings of failure.

Turning Crisis into Opportunity

One of the most empowering ways to approach a crisis is by viewing it as an opportunity for transformation. This doesn't mean minimizing the pain or difficulty of the situation, but recognizing that adversity often serves as a catalyst for growth, change, and self-discovery.

- Learning from Failure: Crises often involve some form of failure or setback. While these moments can be painful, they offer invaluable lessons that can shape your future success. Reflect on what the crisis is teaching you—whether it's about your relationships, career choices, or personal habits—and use those insights to improve.

- Reevaluating Priorities: Crises often force us to reassess our priorities and values. What truly matters to you? Are there areas of your life where you've been neglecting your well-being or goals? Use the adversity as a chance to realign your life with what's most important, shedding unnecessary distractions or pressures that no longer serve you.

- Emerging Stronger: The ultimate goal of handling crisis with grace and strength is not just survival but transformation. Each crisis you face is an opportunity to develop deeper emotional resilience, sharpen your decision-making skills, and strengthen your character. By embracing these challenges, you emerge not only stronger but more capable of facing future adversities with confidence.

The masculine approach to adversity has evolved from mere physical endurance to a more nuanced balance of emotional resilience, decisive action, and vulnerability. Facing personal and professional crises with grace and strength means acknowledging your emotions, acting with clarity, and turning challenges into opportunities for growth. True strength lies not in avoiding hardship but in confronting it with a mindset that is both courageous and adaptable, ultimately leading to a more empowered, resilient version of yourself.

CONCLUSION

As we stand at the intersection of tradition and modernity, masculinity is undergoing a profound transformation. The rigid, one-dimensional image of what it means to be a man no longer fits the complexities of the modern world. In a rapidly changing society, men are being called to redefine their roles—not by abandoning strength, but by expanding it to include emotional intelligence, vulnerability, and a deeper sense of purpose. The future of masculinity depends on this evolution, a shift toward a more holistic, balanced, and empowered form of manhood.

The journey through this book has explored various facets of this evolving masculine identity: from redefining traditional roles and breaking free from limiting stereotypes, to mastering emotional intelligence, vulnerability, and finding personal purpose. It has shown that strength is not diminished by sensitivity, nor is power undermined by vulnerability. In fact, the true power of masculinity lies in its capacity to adapt, grow, and integrate both strength and softness, independence and connection, ambition and compassion.

The future of masculinity is about embracing change without losing the foundational values that make men strong, responsible, and dependable. Integrity, honor, and discipline remain as essential as ever, but they must now be infused with empathy, self-awareness, and adaptability. A man's worth is no longer measured solely by his ability to provide or protect in the traditional sense, but also by how he navigates the emotional and relational landscapes of his life, how he connects with others, and how he contributes to the greater good.

As men evolve into more empowered versions of themselves, they leave behind a powerful legacy. This legacy is not built on traditional markers of success—wealth, power, or status—but on the impact they have on those around them. Empowered masculinity is about lifting others up, inspiring change, and leaving the world better than it was before. It is about being the kind of man who leads with compassion, acts with integrity, and lives with purpose.

The future of masculinity is bright. It is a future where men are free to express the full range of their humanity—strong, sensitive, driven, caring, and purposeful. It is a future where men are no longer confined by outdated expectations but are empowered to forge their own paths. By embracing this evolution, men can not only enrich their own lives but contribute to a more just, compassionate, and equitable world for all.

The Path to Empowered Masculinity is about more than just personal transformation. It is a movement, a shift in the collective consciousness of what it means to be a man. Every step forward in this journey—whether through emotional growth, deeper relationships, or a stronger sense of purpose—contributes to a future where masculinity is defined by its ability to evolve with integrity. This is the new power of manhood, and it is one that every man has the potential to embody.

References

Books and Articles on Masculinity

- Kimmel, M. S. (2008). *Guyland: The Perilous World Where Boys Become Men.* Harper.
- Bly, R. (1990). *Iron John: A Book About Men.* Da Capo Press.
- Connell, R. W. (2005). *Masculinities.* University of California Press.
- Peterson, J. B. (2018). *12 Rules for Life: An Antidote to Chaos.* Random House Canada.
- Katz, J. (2013). *The Macho Paradox: Why Some Men Hurt Women and How All Men Can Help.* Sourcebooks.

Emotional Intelligence and Sensitivity

- Goleman, D. (1995). *Emotional Intelligence: Why It Can Matter More Than IQ.* Bantam Books.
- Brown, B. (2015). *Daring Greatly: How the Courage to Be Vulnerable Transforms the Way We Live, Love, Parent, and Lead.* Avery.
- Bradberry, T., & Greaves, J. (2009). *Emotional Intelligence 2.0.* TalentSmart.

Purpose and Personal Growth

- Sinek, S. (2009). *Start With Why: How Great Leaders Inspire Everyone to Take Action.* Portfolio.
- Clear, J. (2018). *Atomic Habits: An Easy & Proven Way to Build Good Habits & Break Bad Ones.* Avery.

- Frankl, V. E. (2006). *Man's Search for Meaning.* Beacon Press.
- Robbins, A. (2001). *Awaken the Giant Within: How to Take Immediate Control of Your Mental, Emotional, Physical and Financial Destiny!* Free Press.

Mental Health and Crisis Management

- Hari, J. (2018). *Lost Connections: Uncovering the Real Causes of Depression – and the Unexpected Solutions.* Bloomsbury.
- Maté, G. (2003). *When the Body Says No: The Cost of Hidden Stress.* Wiley.
- Siegel, D. J. (2012). *The Mindful Brain: Reflection and Attunement in the Cultivation of Well-Being.* W.W. Norton & Company.
- Miller, I. W., & Rollnick, S. (2012). *Motivational Interviewing: Helping People Change.* The Guilford Press.

Relationships and Communication

- Gottman, J., & Silver, N. (2015). *The Seven Principles for Making Marriage Work: A Practical Guide from the Country's Foremost Relationship Expert.* Harmony.
- Perel, E. (2017). *The State of Affairs: Rethinking Infidelity.* Harper.
- Chapman, G. (1992). *The Five Love Languages: How to Express Heartfelt Commitment to Your Mate.* Northfield Publishing.

Balancing Career, Family, and Growth

- Ferriss, T. (2007). *The 4-Hour Workweek: Escape 9–5, Live Anywhere, and Join the New Rich.* Crown Publishing.
- Covey, S. R. (1989). *The 7 Habits of Highly Effective People: Powerful Lessons in Personal Change.* Free Press.
- Newport, C. (2016). *Deep Work: Rules for Focused Success in a Distracted World.* Grand Central Publishing.

Spirituality and Masculinity

- Tolle, E. (2004). *The Power of Now: A Guide to Spiritual Enlightenment.* New World Library.
- Rohr, R. (2011). *Falling Upward: A Spirituality for the Two Halves of Life.* Jossey-Bass.
- Campbell, J. (1949). *The Hero with a Thousand Faces.* Princeton University Press.

About the Author

James A. Smith is the acclaimed author of *The Path to Empowered Masculinity: Mastering Strength, Sensitivity, and Purpose in a Changing World* and *Mastering Retirement: 20 Proven Strategies for Lasting Wealth, Happiness, and Fulfillment*. With a focus on personal development, leadership, and emotional intelligence, James is passionate about inspiring individuals to live fulfilling lives defined by purpose and balance.

Drawing from a wealth of experience and a deep understanding of human behavior and societal dynamics, James blends practical strategies with meaningful insights to help readers navigate life's challenges and opportunities. His work empowers people to embrace their strengths, foster meaningful connections, and lead lives of intentional growth and resilience.

Disclaimer

The information provided in this book, The Path to Empowered Masculinity: Mastering Strength, Sensitivity, and Purpose in a Changing World, is intended for educational and informational purposes only. It is not a substitute for professional advice, whether medical, psychological, financial, or otherwise.

The author and publisher disclaim any liability arising from the use or application of the concepts, strategies, or techniques discussed in this book. Readers are encouraged to seek appropriate professional consultation or advice for their specific circumstances.

The views expressed in this book are based on the author's research, experience, and opinions. They are not intended to reflect universal truths or to replace individual judgment. Any references to third-party sources or materials are included for informational purposes and do not constitute endorsements.

By reading this book, you acknowledge and accept that the author and publisher are not responsible for any outcomes or consequences resulting from your reliance on the information presented.

Legal Notice

This book, The Path to Empowered Masculinity: Mastering Strength, Sensitivity, and Purpose in a Changing World, and all content contained within, is provided "as is" without any warranties or guarantees of any kind, express or implied. The author and publisher disclaim all liability for any direct, indirect, incidental, or consequential damages resulting from the use of, or inability to use, the information or ideas presented in this book.

The content is intended solely for informational and educational purposes. It is not a substitute for professional advice in any field, including but not limited to medical, psychological, financial, or legal matters. Readers should consult appropriate professionals for advice specific to their individual circumstances.

All trademarks, service marks, and product names mentioned in this book are the property of their respective owners. Their inclusion does not imply any affiliation with or endorsement by the author or publisher.

The author and publisher have made every effort to ensure the accuracy and completeness of the information contained in this book at the time of publication. However, they assume no responsibility for errors, omissions, or changes in the information over time.

By purchasing or reading this book, you agree to indemnify and hold harmless the author, publisher, and any associated parties from any claims, losses, or damages arising from your use of the content provided.

This book is protected under copyright law. Unauthorized reproduction, distribution, or use of any part of this book without prior written consent from the author is strictly prohibited.